THE FIFTEEN MINUTE HOUR
Practical Therapeutic Interventions in Primary Care

THE FIFTEEN MINUTE HOUR
Practical Therapeutic Interventions in Primary Care

MARIAN R. STUART, Ph.D.

JOSEPH A. LIEBERMAN III, M.D., M.P.H.

THIRD EDITION

SAUNDERS
An Imprint of Elsevier Science
Philadelphia London New York St. Louis Sydney Toronto

SAUNDERS
An Imprint of Elsevier Science

The Curtis Center
Independence Square West
Philadelphia, PA 19106

Notice

Pharmacology is an ever-changing field. Standard safety precautions must be followed, but as new research and clinical experience broaden our knowledge, changes in treatment and drug therapy may become necessary or appropriate. Readers are advised to check the most current product information provided by the manufacturer of each drug to be administered to verify the recommended dose, the method and duration of administration, and contraindications. It is the responsibility of the licensed prescriber, relying on experience and knowledge of the patient, to determine dosages and the best treatment for each individual patient. Neither the publisher nor the editor assumes any liability for any injury and/or damage to persons or property arising from this publication.

Previous editions copyrighted 1986, 1993 by Marian R. Stuart and Joseph A. Lieberman III

THE FIFTEEN MINUTE HOUR: Practical Therapeutic Interventions in Primary Care, ed. 3

International Standard Book Number 0–7216–9593–0

Acquisitions Editor: Elizabeth M. Fathman
Publishing Services Manager: Patricia Tannian
Book Design Manager: Gail Morey Hudson
Cover Designer: Teresa Breckwoldt

KO/FF

Printed in the United States of America

Last digit is the print number: 9   8   7   6   5   4   3   2   1

Foreword

Today, perhaps more than ever before, stress plays a role in everyone's life. It affects daily activities, influences the way symptoms are perceived, and detracts from quality of life. Our responsibility as personal physicians is to help our patients manage this stress.

Medicine's earlier preoccupation with a disease-oriented model of health care gave too little recognition to the role that emotions, expectations, fears, and stress play in everyday life. Modern primary care involves a more comprehensive approach to the patient, incorporating biological and psychosocial parameters. Biopsychosocial medicine is an accurate but unwieldy term to describe comprehensive primary care. Primary care recognizes the patient's total life situation and the way psychological and social stress may be contributing to the patient's symptoms.

A primary care physician who is locked into the biological model is much less effective than one who appropriately incorporates the psychological and social aspects of health care. The mind-body approach to medicine is not a dichotomy but a dualism that promotes improved patient care and views the doctor-patient relationship as a complex interaction involving emotional, relational, and belief systems.

Psychotherapy is the term used to describe the treatment of behavioral disturbances employing verbal and nonverbal communication techniques. Primary care physicians use supportive psychotherapy with almost every patient, reinforcing a patient's defenses and relieving symptoms without probing deep psychological conflicts or altering the basic personality. Psychotherapy is not as ominous and difficult as many people believe. It is often most effective when given frequently in small doses by a physician who knows the patient well and enjoys the trust that comes from a long relationship.

This book focuses on psychotherapeutic techniques that every primary care physician can use to care more effectively for patients. Stuart and Lieberman demonstrate in a pragmatic and efficient manner how to incorporate psychotherapy into a busy medical practice. The BATHE technique described in Chapter 6 allows the physician to incorporate the principal features of psychosocial medicine into the patient interview and achieve a better outcome than that obtained by physicians stuck in the disease-oriented model.

Of particular value is the attention paid to listening skills and the importance of empathy, compassion, and respect. Effective communication depends much more on our ability to be good listeners than on what we say to patients. Truly listening to a person is a form of respect, and respect for the patient is an essential ingredient in developing trust and being able to "care with caring." Patients must believe that we value their comments and opinions before they will trust us with information of a personal nature.

A welcome addition to this third edition is the chapter on psychopharmacology, which focuses on the role of pharmacotherapy as an adjunct to behavioral intervention. The use of herbs is included as well as the traditional medications. Depression is a common problem, and patients frequently have a variety of somatic symptoms. Treatment is most effective when psychotherapy is used along with medication. A primary care physician needs specific training to be able to recognize and manage depression in its early stages. Physicians trained in the biopsychosocial model are best prepared to recognize and treat this disorder before it results in significant morbidity or mortality. The identification of potentially serious disease in its early, undifferentiated stage is one of the most difficult and challenging tasks in medicine.

Robert E. Rakel, M.D.
Professor
Department of Family and Community Medicine
Baylor College of Medicine
Houston, Texas

Preface

The publication of this third edition of *The Fifteen Minute Hour* by Elsevier Science is a source of great satisfaction to us. The purpose of the book has not changed since the appearance of the first edition in 1986. It is to convince you that by routinely incorporating therapeutic interventions into primary care practice, you can solve or even prevent many problems. During the years since publication of the first edition, many things have changed. In earlier editions we speculated about a number of mind-body connections that have since been substantiated by research. The increase in terrorism in the United States and around the world has compromised people's basic sense of safety. Evidenced-based medicine, electronic communications, cost control, cultural diversity, and other societal trends have affected the delivery of medical care. In spite of all these changes, the importance of the practitioner-patient relationship remains a constant. The approaches described in this text are designed not only to enhance the therapeutic relationship, but also to make your practice more productive and pleasurable. The book has grown out of our combined 60+ years of clinical practice and our experience in training residents, practicing physicians, nurse practitioners, and other primary care providers in the art of therapeutic talk. In the 15 years since the publication of the first edition of *The Fifteen Minute Hour*, we have heard from many enthusiastic practitioners in the United States, Canada, Australia, the United Kingdom, Denmark, Malta, Korea, and elsewhere who have assimilated our techniques into their practices. We were ecstatic when the second edition was translated into Japanese because this attested to the multicultural relevance of our techniques. The overwhelming consensus is that the strategies work: patients respond, practitioners save time, provider-patient relationships become richer, and everyone feels a little less stressed out.

This book is not a comprehensive text on psychiatry in primary care. Many good books about that subject are available. It is also not a text on psychoanalysis or long-term psychotherapy. Although our techniques will certainly increase your ability to recognize and treat emotional problems, often at an early and manageable state, we are invested primarily in enhancing your ability to diagnose and manage common, treatable emotional conditions that result from the stress of living in the twenty-first century. Therefore this is a book about incorporating useful knowledge from psychology and psychotherapy into medical practice to become more effective in dealing with the emotional overlay or underlay of problems patients bring to the primary care practitioner.

When *The Fifteen Minute Hour* was first published, the importance of addressing the psychological issues related to the patient's health status were not seen as critical. Max Planck has been quoted as explaining that "a new scientific truth does not triumph by convincing its opponents and making them see the light, but rather because its opponents eventually die, and a new generation grows up that is familiar with it." You are our new generation. We hope that you will master our simple techniques to deal effectively with the psychological dimension of patient care. If you already focus on patients' psychosocial problems or would like to do so more efficiently, this book will provide you with theoretical background material that will help you understand universal principles. We will point out what actually works in practice to improve patients' functioning. Furthermore, we will provide specific suggestions, approaches to therapeutic interventions, and particular phrases that we have developed, practiced, taught, and tested for over 20 years. Preliminary research suggests that our approach improves practitioner-patient relationships[1] and patient satisfaction[2] without adding significantly to the length of the visit.[3]

Our way is not necessarily the only true, good, or beautiful way to make therapeutic interventions, but it is a pragmatic and flexible approach that is easily learned, and it works! Also, it is designed to fit into a regular office visit of 15 minutes or less without requiring lengthy therapy sessions.

We strongly recommend that you read this book from beginning to end. Early chapters provide the theoretical background and rationale, and subsequent chapters focus on putting this knowledge into action. In essence, this is a how-to book. We aim to help you develop skills that will benefit both you and your patient. We provide some effective tools for use in your practice, and we explain exactly how to use them. These tools require less investment of time and energy than you might imagine.

There are many schools of therapy. We are not preaching a dogma, nor do we have the need to establish a true religion in this area. We are quite comfortable with practical eclecticism because it works, and primary care practitioners desperately need techniques that work. We invite you to apply our techniques and empirically confirm their usefulness for yourself. In essence, we are saying, "Try it, you'll like it."

John Godfrey Saxe, a Vermont lawyer and humorist, wrote "The Blind Men and the Elephant"[4] over 100 years ago. This poem was based on an Indian tale thought to date back thousands of years. It still seems most applicable.

> It was six men of Indostan
>   To learning much inclined,
> Who went to see the Elephant
>   (Though all of them were blind)
> That each by observation
>   Might satisfy his mind.
>
> The First approached the Elephant,
>   And happening to fall
> Against his broad and sturdy side,
>   At once began to bawl:
> "God bless me! but the Elephant
>   Is very like a wall!"
>
> The Second, feeling of the tusk,
>   Cried, "Ho! what have we here

So very round and smooth and sharp?
     To me 'tis mighty clear
This wonder of an Elephant
     Is very like a spear!"

The Third approached the animal,
     And happening to take
The squirming trunk within his hands,
     Thus boldly up and spake:
"I see," quoth he, "the Elephant
     Is very like a snake!"

The Fourth reached out an eager hand,
     And felt about the knee
"What most this wondrous beast is like
     Is mighty plain," quoth he;
' "Tis clear enough the Elephant
     Is very like a tree!"

The Fifth who chanced to touch the ear,
     Said: "E'en the blindest man
Can tell what this resembles most;
     Deny the fact who can,
This marvel of an Elephant
     Is very like a fan!"

The Sixth no sooner had begun
     About the beast to grope
Than, seizing on the swinging tail
     That fell within his cope,
"I see," quoth he, "the Elephant
     Is very like a rope!"

And so these men of Indostan
     Disputed loud and long,
Each in his own opinion
     Exceeding stiff and strong,
Though each was partly in the right,
     And all were in the wrong!

Different schools of psychology and psychiatry view the patient and the patient's problems from different perspectives. Each provides a small piece of useful insight. Collectively these fragments form a practical armamentarium with which to reduce patients' suffering, prevent physical and psychological illnesses they might develop, and help them to structure satisfying lives for themselves and their loved ones.

In writing this book, we have tried to present a coherent whole. Each chapter builds on the previous one, and illustrative clinical examples appear throughout the text. The case material, including a dozen new examples, is based entirely on actual encounters, although we have changed names and altered some details to guarantee patients' confidentiality. In revising the text for this edition, we have considered the many thoughtful critiques and reviews of *The Fifteen Minute Hour* and have clarified and expanded important sections. In addition to providing new case material, concepts, and techniques, we have included a chapter on the use of psychotropic medication.

In Chapter 1 we discuss current trends in the delivery of health care, the outmoded "medical model," and the need to use a new structure that integrates George Engel's biopsychosocial model with an awareness of current sociological, political, and economic realities. Chapter 2 details patients' reactions to stress and provides a theoretical basis for the effectiveness of the type of interventions we are promoting. We bring together research findings from a variety of sources, some of which may be new to you, and try to establish a strong foundation. In Chapter 3 we discuss the qualifications and natural proclivities that enable primary care practitioners to make effective therapeutic interventions.

Chapter 4 presents, from a variety of viewpoints, the actual elements that induce the positive changes attributed to psychotherapy. We discuss the elements common to all schools of psychotherapy and introduce several new concepts to simplify the process of inducing positive change. Chapter 5 looks at the differences between the type of therapy we are advocating and the therapy generally provided by traditional mental health practitioners. The second part of this chapter falls into the "how-to" category, as we suggest ways to take advantage of these differences and discuss the time and procedure for making referrals.

Chapter 6 explains how to structure the basic therapeutic intervention. Chapters 7 and 8 provide a rich variety of techniques that can be used in brief, follow-up counseling sessions with patients. Chapter 9 describes the use of pharmacological agents to enhance basic psychological treatment and improve patients' ability to function. Chapters 10 and 11 provide clear directions for implementing our proposals, including what to do, how, when, and with whom. Throughout the book we have expanded material related to anxiety, depression, grief, posttraumatic stress, bulimia, and dealing with children and teens. At the request of a number of practitioners, we have added new material related to behavioral medicine. Chapter 12 projects our vision of what is possible for primary care practice given widespread acceptance and application of these ideas.

We hope you will enjoy reading *The Fifteen Minute Hour*. Please have fun with it. Your patients will thank you many times over.

Marian R. Stuart, Ph.D.
Joseph A. Lieberman III, M.D.

REFERENCES

1. Kallerup, H. *Patients' and doctors' considerations about using communications strategies.* Proceedings from the 24th Annual Meeting of the North American Primary Care Research Group, Vancouver, BC, Canada, Nov 3–6, 1996.
2. Jones, K., Major, G., & Marvel K. *Counseling patients for lifestyle change: a comparison of two methods.* Proceedings from the Society of Teachers of Family Medicine, Seattle, Wash., May, 1998.
3. Dickey, J.H., Woodhouse, W.M., Stephens, S., & Solbrig, R. Impact of the BATHE technique on appointment duration and patient and provider satisfaction. Submitted for publication to *Family Medicine*, 2001.
4. Saxe, J.G. *Clever Stories of Many Nations: Rendered in Rhyme.* Boston: Ticknor & Fields, 1865.

Acknowledgments

We wish to recognize and express appreciation to the many people who made meaningful contributions to this book and earlier editions. We would first like to thank the following physicians: Maria Auletta, M.D.; Hana Chaim, D.O.; Alicia Dermer, M.D.; Steven Frank, D.O.; Joan Gopin, M.D.; Patricia Janku, M.D.; Naomi Kolb, M.D.; Paula M. Krauser, M.D., M.A.; Ronald Lau, M.D.; Yves Morency, M.D.; Jay D. Patel, M.D.; Jean Plover, M.D.; Jamie L. Reedy, M.D., M.P.H.; Andrew Sachere, M.D.; Yasser Soliman, M.D.; Roger Thompson, M.D.; Harvey Weingarten, M.D.; and Tanya Zaremba (medical student, class of 2002) for practicing our methods and contributing experiential clinical material. We would also like to acknowledge our colleagues Robert C. Like, M.D.; David E. Swee, M.D.; Lynne A. Schwenzer, M.H.S.A.; and Alfred F. Tallia for their continuing support and encouragement. Special thanks to Beatrix Hamm, M.D.; John F. Clabby, Ph.D.; and Afton L. Hassett, Psy.D., for their research and editorial assistance. Finally, we would like to thank Robin Covington, Enid Cruz, Louise Ignosia, Ellen Justice, Sara Schlessinger, Judy DiMichele, Dolores Moran, Leanne Mallet-Prevost, Joan Roberts, and Diane Wolf, without whose skill and support our work could not have been completed.

Marian R. Stuart, Ph.D.
Joseph A. Lieberman III, M.D.

Contents

The New Medical Model for the Twenty-First Century: Focusing on the Totality of the Body-Mind

Amerian medicine, although continuously undergoing evolution, now faces changes the magnitude of which have never before been encountered. The dramatic proliferation of knowledge in general; the effects of burgeoning technology; the information accessible on the Internet; sociological changes within the community that encourage wellness and self-help programs; redirection of financial resources, with material constraints imposed on both the public and private sectors; and increased personal longevity with its concomitant chronic illnesses are only some of the responsible factors. Individually and collectively, these phenomena continue to reshape the system of American health care delivery.

Responding to this level of ferment can be distressing, forbidding, and uncomfortable for practitioners. At the same time, it can be seen as challenging, fortuitous, and, in some ways, refreshing. Finding successful ways of adapting to changing circumstances becomes the primary task. The practitioner who wishes to endure and prosper is faced with the need to acquire new skills and rethink ideas that are currently being challenged. It is critical to meet the patients' emerging needs. The ability to clearly comprehend the scope of these needs is the central issue.

We know that the first step in solving any problem is to identify it. The simple recognition of a situation as a problem alters it. This book is largely devoted to looking at the practitioner-patient relationship and the patients' needs from a somewhat untraditional perspective. We hope in this way to identify problems that heretofore may not have been considered by the traditionally trained physician. It is precisely in the resolution of these problems that the contemporary practitioner will gain the skills needed to practice medicine effectively in this new, and at times difficult, climate of health care delivery. There is a considerable body of literature demonstrating that patients encountered by primary care practitioners commonly present with a psychiatric or at least a behavioral problem as the reason for seeking care.[1,2]

Even in those instances where a patient is seen for an obvious biomedical problem, there frequently is an emotional overlay that needs to be addressed if the patient is to receive optimal care. One of the strengths of primary care practice is the diversity of patient problems. This also gives rise to profound challenges, particularly regarding the behavioral and, in more extreme cases, the psychiatric aspects of this type of practice.

Compounding the difficulty of this situation is the recognition that the primary care practitioner is the backbone of America's mental health system, providing a larger percentage of mental health services than do specialists in mental and addictive disorders.[3] In many communities the primary care practitioner is the only professional with training in mental health available to patients.[3] The delivery of effective health care requires a cadre of practitioners who are capable of providing appropriate psychiatric interventions to diminish the suffering of their patients. One of the most enlightened ways to do this is by addressing the sources of their distress and not just the effects.[4]

LIMITS OF THE TRADITIONAL DISEASE-ORIENTED MEDICAL MODEL

To understand better why contemporary clinicians need to acquire new skills, we might start by looking at how these practitioners were trained (how they acquired their current skills). Until recently, traditional medicine has concerned itself almost exclusively with the biomedical model of illness. Medical education has perpetuated this approach with its overwhelming emphasis on tertiary care and bench research. Few professors (the role models for the next generations of clinicians) ever encounter the undifferentiated patient population that is the daily fare of the generalist. The halls of academe have little appreciation of the role of the primary care provider who practices at the interface of the biomedical, behavioral, and social sciences. The academic model creates a structure for examining, classifying, and treating disease. In the process, this pathogenic orientation creates a dichotomous classification of people as either having or not having a disease. Diseases are viewed almost in isolation from their patient victims. This reductionistic approach, which literally separates the patient from the disease, has been the working model in our systems of medical education and health care delivery. It is the disease that is on center stage, and efforts are directed mainly toward categorizing it from the appropriate etiological and therapeutic perspectives. The disease is the *raison d'être* for the doctor-patient encounter, and thus, in most instances, it dictates an acute care setting.

To arrive at the proper etiology, and thereby establish the proper therapy, the reductionistic approach is also used in clinical decision making. Diseases are traditionally put into large classifications and then gradually subclassified until the specific disease entity is identified. Further, it is assumed that each disease has a specific cause for which treatment, in one form or another, is generally available. Frequently, the choice among chemical, surgical, radiological, or other treatment must be made, but it is always with the intention of somehow counteracting the cause of the pathological condition and thereby changing the natural course of the disease. The main function of the traditional physician has been to direct this process for the patient and to prescribe an appropriate therapy after an etiological diagnosis has been established.

This type of clinical reasoning lends itself particularly well to the generalist's need for a system with which to approach an undifferentiated patient population. By this, we mean the need for a model that will enable the primary care provider to deal effectively with a waiting room full of patients who have varying and unorganized signs, symptoms, and problems. Frequently, these patients have few external clues as to the nature of their particular problem. Categorization, followed by subcategorization, and then subsubcategorization, efficiently leads one from these broad-based, frequently ill-defined presenting problems to a manageable diagnostic entity that is then amenable to a specific therapeutic intervention. The practitioner is thus able to sort through a variety of data in an efficiently organized fashion and arrive at a meaningful conclusion that shapes a specific action.

There is a real problem with the above scenario. Although it certainly works in clarifying issues for the practitioner, we agree with George Engel[5] that the following is true:

> The crippling flaw of the model is that it does not include the patient and his attributes as a person, as a human being. The biomedical model can make provision neither for the person as a whole nor for data of a psychological or social nature, for the reductionism and mind-body dualism on which the model is predicated requires that these must first be reduced to physico-chemical terms before they can have meaning. Hence, the very essence of medical practice perforce remains "art" and beyond the reach of science (p. 536).

It would seem that the biopsychosocial sum is greater than the sum of the biomedical parts. In spite of the fact that it may not add up properly, the biomedical model is still the preeminent way in which contemporary American medicine is practiced. A better understanding of this process can be achieved by examining its application in its most common form, the typical office encounter.

NATURE OF THE OFFICE ENCOUNTER

Under ordinary circumstances, patients arrive at the practitioner's office with a symptom or collection of symptoms. The clinician goes through a series of physical assessments and laboratory and other evaluations to arrive at a working hypothesis concerning the cause of the symptoms and the nature, therefore, of the disease. After developing a differential diagnosis and listing numerous disease entities that might account for the symptoms, the clinician uses the available data to rule out the most serious ailments and eventually arrives at a diagnosis that provides a label for the patient's condition. The appropriate therapy is then prescribed. Since this is commonly a pharmacological agent, the prescription will now be generated. In fact, issuing the prescription consistently marks the end of the encounter. If no pathological cause can be established for the patient's symptoms, the diagnosis is frequently made that they are some manifestation of a behavioral or emotional disorder. Again, a prescription will be given to relieve the symptoms. Now, however, the clinician will more likely order a psychotherapeutic agent. Nevertheless, the encounter is still terminated in the same fashion. The implication that every disease must have a specific cause and that this cause can usually be treated pharmacologically is central to the process. If a definite cause for the illness cannot be ascertained, then at least the symptoms can be treated, also pharmacologically.

The office encounter is now almost complete. The patient only has to pay for the visit or sign the insurance form attesting to having received specific services.

Tension Between the Scientific Method and Patients' Needs

It is regrettable that this entire scenario frequently meets the needs of the practitioner far better than those of the patient. Perhaps this is the central problem: Patients arrive at the clinician's office knowing only that they do not feel well and have symptoms. After a series of maneuvers and studies, patients are informed of a likely cause for their symptoms. If this is responsive to a specific therapy, they will be fortunate enough to have their symptoms relieved and be considered cured. The practitioner is gratified that the patient can, in fact, be treated, and the patient is satisfied and grateful, since the particular problem has been dealt with effectively. Far more commonly, however, the patient's symptoms are part of a much bigger picture. Patients are complex, multidimensional human beings, and they bring a variety of problems to the clinician, some of which are quite obvious, whereas others take the form of hidden agendas. I.R. McWhinney[6] suggests that if the "patient is fortunate, he will find a physician who will meet these needs as well as providing the best of technical care." If the underlying reasons for a patient's visit are to be discerned, the clinician needs to be a perceptive student of human nature. Instead, if the practitioner simply focuses on the obvious organic aspects of the presentation, this unidimensional view may prevent an accurate diagnosis of the patient's real problems.

The presenting problem (which the practitioner can frequently handle with little difficulty) may not be the main reason for the patient's visit. A substantial body of literature shows that people visit clinicians not only for relief of organic disorders, but also because of life stress, psychiatric disorders, social isolation, and informational needs.[7] Even those patients who are fortunate enough to have their symptoms relieved by the clinician's intervention may find this insufficient to meet all their other needs. For example, recent studies suggest that many patients believe spirituality plays an important role in their lives and that there is a positive correlation between a patient's spirituality or religious commitment and health outcomes; patients would like practitioners to consider these factors in their medical care.[8] If, on the other hand, patients have the misfortune of not even having their symptoms relieved and are informed that, in fact, it is "only your nerves that are causing your symptoms," they become subject to the stigma that the explanation implies. All too frequently, they are left with a therapy that will relieve their most obvious symptoms but will not treat the underlying condition. By "turning off" the symptom (which is a signal that something is wrong), the clinician removes the evidence without addressing the problem. By analogy, if we were to turn off the bell on our telephone, we would never know when someone was calling and would not be able to respond.

INTERRELATIONSHIP BETWEEN PHYSICAL AND PSYCHOLOGICAL HEALTH

The use of the reductionistic approach can be very valuable at times, particularly when a specific physical malady can explain the patient's symptoms. However, if the clinician is to be a true healer, this approach is far too limited for dealing with patient needs. A whole body of recent research substantiates the inadequacy of the traditional biological approach in the evaluation of symptoms.[7,9] These investigations indicate conclusively that the soma does not function in a vacuum but rather that the psyche and the soma are so closely related that imbalances in either one can produce symptoms or disease in the other.

Indeed, studies devoted to stress-related disorders have increased geometrically. For example, a patient's psychological response to diagnosis or treatment of cancer can be related to the course of the disease.[10] S. Greer, T. Morris, and K.W. Pettingale[11] found that women diagnosed with breast cancer who express anger and hostility have a better prognosis than those who passively and helplessly accept their disease. D. Spiegel and his colleagues[12] were amazed to find that women with breast cancer who were in support groups not only had a much better quality of life (as had been expected) but also survived significantly longer than women in the control group. Since this initial study, much similar research has been conducted, leading reviewers to conclude that emotional processes can affect cancer progression, quality of life, and survival.[13–15]

Effects of Stress on the Immune System

R.W. Bartrop and his colleagues[16] were the first to report on the mechanisms involved in the well-known mortality risk following bereavement. A prospective study published in the *Journal of the American Medical Association* replicated their study by monitoring the immune system of husbands of women with breast cancer and found a highly significant suppression of lymphocyte function to specific antigens within one month of the spouse's death.[17] This suppression lasted for 14 months after bereavement and was not due to pre-existing conditions. The investigators concluded that "suppressed immunity following the death of a spouse may be related to the increased morbidity and mortality associated with bereavement" (p. 374).[17] In another study, published in the *New England Journal of Medicine*, psychological stress was found not only to increase the risk of contracting an infectious respiratory disease but also to have a dose-related effect.[18]

Over the last 20 years, findings from the field of psychoneuroimmunology (PNI) have provided insight into the possible mechanisms involved in the relationship between psychological factors and the pathogenesis of disease. The following findings have been cited by R. Ader and colleagues[19] as the most compelling evidence for the bidirectional communication between the nervous and immune systems: (1) Nerve endings can be found in the tissues of the immune system. (2) Central nervous system (CNS) changes alter immune response, and an immune response alters CNS activity. (3) An immune response alters hormone and neurotransmitter levels and vice versa. (4) Lymphocytes are able to produce neurotransmitters and hormones. (5) Psychological factors may render one vulnerable to the progression of autoimmune disease, infectious disease, and cancer. (6) Immunological reactivity can be influenced by stress, hypnosis, and classical conditioning.

Other Body-Mind Interactions

J.M. Weiss[20] describes numerous experimental studies leading to an increased understanding of the mechanisms involved in the development of peptic ulcers and other gastrointestinal pathological conditions. In fact, as early as 1917, Trendelenburg demonstrated that embedded within the wall of the gut was a self-contained, self-regulating nervous system that could function on its own, without the help of the brain or the spinal cord.[21] The gut, in short, has a mind of its own. Studies of the pathophysiological links between behavioral factors and cardiovascular disease and other life-threatening illnesses are also proliferating.[22] For example, depression has been shown to be a risk factor for cardiac disease.[23-26] Other studies focus on the role of psychosocial influences on morbidity and mortality after a myocardial infarction.[27-31] Three recent literature reviews support a strong relationship of negative emotions (depression, anxiety, anger), life stress, and inadequate social support to coronary heart disease.[32-34] Although the findings support the notion of a causal relationship, conclusive proof is still pending. Instead, these psychological factors should be considered important (modifiable) risk factors. However, if the psyche and the soma were not integrally related, none of these effects would occur.

It is not our intention in this chapter to provide an exhaustive review of the literature. Instead, our wish is to heighten awareness and indicate the importance of incorporating these understandings into the day-to-day practice of medicine. In his introduction to Norman Cousins's *The Healing Heart*, the cardiologist Bernard Lown[35] wrote the following:

Although most physicians would not deny that many variables, including psychological factors, influence disease, these are regarded as secondary and largely irrelevant once the basic cause is discovered. For example, when streptococcal upper-respiratory infections are controlled, psychological factors in a child's rheumatic fever are not given serious consideration. . . . Similarly, some physicians would maintain that once the biology of cancer is comprehended, the psychological factors that may govern its progress or modulate its anxiety and pain become but an irrelevant script on ancient scrolls.

The most immutable fact of life is death. It will never be annulled by artificial organs or scientific progress. The days of a human being will ever be finite, and disease and pain will always stalk life's journey. The patient will always require care, sympathetic judgment, and healing. The physician will never be relieved of the responsibility to assuage pain, promote comfort, and instill hope. But there is an additional aspect, relating to the patient's psychobiological constitution that has powerful self-regulating and self-healing capacities. In ignoring these intrinsic gifts for self-repair, the physician obstructs the amplification of the efficacy of his own scientific methods and impedes the very process of recovery.

DECLINE OF THE RELEVANCE OF TRADITIONAL MEDICINE

It is regrettable that failure to recognize all that the relationship between the psyche and soma implies—by unwisely relying on the traditional approach—is resulting in meeting ever fewer needs of an enlightened patient population. This has caused a certain public disenchantment with the medical profession and has spurred the growth and proliferation of many self-help and allied programs. If, indeed, a practitioner does not answer a patient's needs, then the patient will seek help elsewhere, even though this decision may ultimately be to the patient's detriment.

Cults, quacks, vitamin megadoses, purges, extreme nutritionalism, and other fads, which are in some ways reminiscent of the Dark Ages, continue to flourish in our society, in many ways spurred by the public's disenchantment with the medical establishment and its inability to meet their individual needs. Alternative medicine (or complementary medicine) is clearly the largest growth industry in health care today.[36] Sixty-nine percent of Americans used some form of alternative medicine in 1998. Use of specific types of complementary medicine in 1998 included relaxation 43%, vitamin therapy 43%, chiropractic 42%, herbal medicine 41%, massage 33%, folk medicine 26%, and homeopathy 11%.[37] Certainly, constructive self-help is a good thing. Programs to reduce stress; improve physical conditioning; do away with drug, alcohol, and cigarette dependency; and maintain ideal height/weight ratios and good physical conditioning are all to be encouraged. Unfortunately, much of the impetus in these various areas has been taken by the lay public and not by the medical profession per se. R.B. Taylor[38] has underscored the need for health care providers, whose scientific knowledge dictates a rational approach that promotes living wisely, to take the lead rather than leaving it to cultism or financial aspirations of alternative interests. Many components of the self-help movement, although constructive, are in fact still another manifestation of public dissatisfaction with the traditional healing arts and their perceived inability to deal with the individual patient and his or her needs.

ECONOMIC CONSIDERATIONS

The restructuring of the financial reimbursement system for medical services provides yet another incentive for contemporary clinicians to rethink the way they practice. Seventy-five percent of American health care costs are borne by government and industry.[39] The major government programs are Medicare (mostly for elderly people) and Medicaid (for the indigent population, poor young children, and unemployable adults). Private health insurance is most commonly provided by large employers and is considered a benefit of employment. The majority of those who do not have health insurance but are employed work for small companies that do not offer this benefit. These employees are also frequently on the lower end of the pay scale. This form of health insurance (government programs for the very young, old, or unemployable population or an employee benefit predominantly offered by large corporations) is unique in Western society and gives rise to many inequities in access to the health care system. The ability to work within this system, while at the same time trying to change it to a more equitable one, is one of the many challenges facing the contemporary practitioner.

Historically, in the United States, the preeminent method of paying physicians has been on a fee-for-service basis. Under this system, a patient typically would present to a physician with an illness, such as appendicitis, and a service, in this instance an appendectomy, would be performed by the physician. A fee would then be collected from the patient or the patient's insurance carrier. With this method, high-tech services are generally compensated better than the so-called cognitive services, although both may involve equivalent time and effort on the physician's part. Such a system, of course, rewards utilization, because there is no payment unless the service is rendered. Likewise, such a system favors more complicated approaches over simpler ones, as well as procedural services over cognitive ones, because in both instances the former type is more liberally rewarded financially.

Other provider payment systems, loosely grouped under the term "managed care," pay the physician or other practitioner a predetermined amount for care provided to a patient or family over a specified period. This form of reimbursement rewards the practitioner who can minimize expenditures (e.g., hospitalization, laboratory, or pharmacy costs) and maximize wellness. This system also rewards conservation of those funds earmarked for payment to other specialists or consultants. The popularity of this sort of reimbursement, however, waxes and wanes. To some it is perceived as rewarding withholding benefits to patients in much the same way as fee-for-service reimbursement encourages and rewards "overtreatment." To date no system has emerged that would build on the advantages offered by each of these competing systems without concurrently running the risk of exacerbating their respective disadvantages. Further complicating this picture is the development of still another career path for primary care providers, that is, the role of hospitalists. These practitioners work largely within the confines of hospitals and care for patients while they are in this setting. Hospitalists are frequently trained in a primary care discipline as generalists. As a result of this training, they are deemed to be well prepared to deal with the multiplicity and variety of problems encountered in hospitalized patients. However, in most instances, they do not have continuity of care practices, at least when it comes to those patients that they treat in their hospitalist role. Nonetheless, these practitioners need to be aware that an impressive and rapidly growing body of literature documents the necessity and cost effectiveness of providing psychological support to patients in hospitals as well as outpatient settings.[40–45]

Regardless of the method of reimbursement, it is interesting to note that patients are frequently the innocent players in these scenarios, since they have little choice and virtually no expertise concerning the services they are to receive. With the proliferation of health care insurance, and various carve-outs, patients also bear little responsibility for the financial consequences of their practitioners' actions. In addition, at least in the fee-for-service environment, clinicians frequently find themselves in the position of being rewarded only if they "do something" and of being pressured by patients who, because they have insurance, want something done! Right or wrong, much of the blame for rapidly rising health costs is laid on this method of reimbursement.

This book presents strategies that will provide effective psychosocial treatment in the context of a standard office practice. These strategies, coupled with good medical practice, should enable the knowledgeable practitioner to maintain a competitive position relative to other practitioners in what is becoming a crowded profession. As Paul Starr[46] bluntly pointed out, "Increasingly, the gains of one physician, or group of physicians, will have to come at the expense of other physicians or providers." Perceptive clinicians must acquire the skills that are needed to flourish in just such a professional environment.

Those of us in the healing professions need to start looking critically at what we do and analyze how well we are providing the services for which the public seeks us out. To deal purely with the physical realm is, in almost all instances, to deal only incompletely with the patient's problems. We must be able to expand somewhat on our ability to meet the patient's needs while at the same time conserving our resources so that we may meet the needs of all our patients.

We need to reexamine what we do and change the model, or paradigm, by which we operate. Thomas Kuhn's observations[47] led him to suggest that there is a cycle determining scientific revolutions that must occur periodically. M.J. Mahoney[48] described Kuhn's contribution very concisely:

> According to Kuhn, "normal science" is a powerful problem-solving machine dedicated to grinding out the rich harvest of experimentation. As the machine becomes more precise and productive, however, there are increasing probabilities of encountering—or more accurately, recognizing—anomalies. These anomalous pieces of information do not fit the paradigm's conceptual categories and/or predictions and they cannot be assimilated without at least adjusting, if not overhauling, the machine.

Research has brought to light phenomena that simply cannot be fit into the traditional biomedical model. Because of the new information that we have acquired about both patients and disease, it would seem that traditional medicine is at that point in Kuhn's cycle where the conceptual categories are in need of a serious overhaul. We must shift, or change, the paradigm in order to build a new structure that accommodates our current understandings and points to a more effective practice. McWhinney[49] summarizes the seven central concepts of the old paradigm of medicine:
1. Patients suffer from diseases that can be categorized.
2. Diseases are independent of the persons suffering from them.
3. Each disease has a specific causal agent.
4. The physician's task is to diagnose and prescribe.
5. The correct disease can be determined through a process of differential diagnosis.
6. The patient is a passive recipient of this process.
7. Mental and physical diseases can be considered separately, except in specific psychosomatic diseases where the mind appears to act on the body.

There are several major limitations in the traditional medical model. McWhinney goes on to discuss three particular anomalies: the illness-disease anomaly, the specific etiology anomaly, and the mind-body anomaly. The first concerns the incidence of illness without disease. Studies of abdominal pain have shown that specific diagnoses were obtained in less than 50% of cases. Headache, chest pain, back pain, and other illnesses often present in the absence of clear-cut, identifiable disease.

The second anomaly concerns the general susceptibility to disease that is evidenced by some individuals. Why is it that 25% of the patients have 75% of the illnesses? If diseases truly had specific etiologies, then it would seem likely that every person would have an even chance of contracting them. However, this is not the case. Subsequent chapters will discuss some factors that make people either more or less vulnerable.

The third anomaly concerns the effects of mind on the body. Factors such as the impact of social isolation and stressful life events on health or the placebo effect cannot be explained using the traditional medical model. In every controlled trial, a percentage of people respond physiologically to an inert substance. The magnitude of the placebo effect varies in every study, but it actually approaches 100% in some instances. Recently, in a study published in the *New England Journal of Medicine*, A. Hrobjartsson and P. Gotzsche[50] concluded that patients given placebos improve at about the same rate as those who receive no treatment. Based on their results, they propose that there is no justification for the use of placebos outside the setting of clinical trials. However, in 27 of the studies even these authors found that placebos had a beneficial effect on *pain*. In an accompanying editorial in that same publication Dr. John Bailar III,[51] emeritus professor from the University of Chicago, generally supports their conclusions although he does admit that he feels their recommendations "may be just a bit too sweeping."

We would respectfully submit that these authors are all missing the point. The difference between treatment and healing has to come from within. The mind, as an organ that processes information (beliefs), interacts with the body by producing chemical changes that initiate chain reactions. Jerome Frank[52] has written a provocative commentary entitled "The Placebo Is Psychotherapy." We wholeheartedly agree.

Perhaps the most important factor in developing a new and more effective medical model is a focus on the process of the practitioner-patient relationship and the patient's interaction with the environment. The role of the practitioner will be increasingly to mobilize the patient's own healing power. Norman Cousins[53] underscores the effectiveness of confidence in the body's recovery potential, involvement in the treatment, and a sense of partnership with the physician as making a major contribution to creating the physiological healing response.

It should be obvious that the old paradigm has, in fact, been overwhelmed and that, if a practitioner is to remain relevant, he or she must change the approach taken toward the patient. This contemporary practitioner must deal with the paradox that has resulted when training dictates the isolation of an illness by a reductionistic approach, yet patients present with multiple needs in which the disease entity may only play a part of varying importance.

DEVELOPING AN INTEGRATED (HOLISTIC) APPROACH BASED ON SCIENTIFIC METHOD

Certainly George Engel's conceptualization of the biopsychosocial model[54] presents an innovative and relevant way in which to apply the tenets of modern biology and the behavioral sciences to a patient encounter. In this way, the biological bases are fully exposed and touched on, while at the same time the psychosocial context is incorporated.

Engel[5] believes, as we do, that the basic organic building blocks—that is, subatomic particles, atoms, molecules, up through cells, tissues, organs, and organisms—are part of a larger system, including the family, community, subculture, and on up through the biosphere. He has further maintained that the systems are interrelated to the degree that an event impacting on any one component has an effect on all other components. He presents clinical examples, such as the stress-related illness of an electrical engineer, that produce events in a community, such as loss of income, failure of businesses, and outward migration of the population. In this example, he also demonstrates the impact of stress on the engineer's organ systems, with the production of such signs and symptoms as lethargy, pain, and nausea. In another example, Engel refers to a case of severe physical and mental retardation caused by radiation-induced mutation. He demonstrates how this impact will, at the subatomic particle level, lead to arrested development in tissues, organs, and systems; cause emotional trauma at the family level; and produce an overall resource strain at the biosphere level.

In both examples, Engel cites many other effects that result from an adverse impact sustained predominantly at just one level in this system. We join him in questioning the wisdom of dissecting out certain levels, such as the cellular, tissue, and organ systems, for study in a reductionistic and isolated fashion. This is a characteristic style of the medical profession, which tends to leave the balance of the effects on the total system to other disciplines.

A massive and evolving body of literature substantiates the anecdotal observations of most practitioners who deal with patients day to day. It has been repeatedly noted that many events that are far removed from the organ and tissue levels will nonetheless have profound effects on components of the system. Therefore, to study and treat these components in the abstract, and only in the biomedical context, is a form of undertreatment that is every bit as damaging to the patient as undertreatment would be in any other form.

Almost a quarter of a century ago, building on the work of George Engel, McWhinney[55] underscored the need to develop a new, more relevant paradigm of medicine, incorporating the following concepts:

1. More attention must be paid to health promotion and disease prevention.
2. We must keep separate disease categories but recognize the effects of interactions and disease susceptibility.
3. We must pay more attention to nonorganic factors, such as environmental and relationship characteristics, when determining the etiology of disease.
4. The role of the physician is to mobilize the patient's own healing powers.
5. Physicians must develop advanced communication skills in order to diagnose and treat patients (rather than diseases).
6. Physicians must develop skills to elicit the meaning of the illness to the patient.
7. The body, mind, and spirit are integrated.

When putting these principles into practice, it is important not only to investigate and integrate the psychosocial aspects of patients' lives into our understanding of their illnesses but also to intervene by supporting our patients and tapping into their own resources in order to optimize outcome.

The traditional reductionistic approach to medical practice has had as its end point an understanding of how a particular disease developed in a given patient. An often-quoted aphorism attributed to Sir William Osler states, "It is much more important to know what sort of patient has a disease than what sort of disease a patient has." Still, that does not tell us exactly what should be done about either the patient or the disease. Our intention is to clearly spell out for the practitioner how to use this information to potentiate a patient's own resources and thereby improve the outcome. The following chapters will discuss practical interventions that can be used to achieve these ends.

SUMMARY

Given the dramatic proliferation in medical knowledge, technology, and costs of care; sociological changes within the community that encourage wellness and self-help programs; and redirection of financial resources to include prospective payment plans, the primary care practitioner is urged to reassess and discard the traditional reductionistic, disease-oriented medical model. The typical office encounter has generally met the needs of the clinician more fully than the multidimensional needs of the patient. Recognizing the interrelationship between physical and psychological health, the true inseparability of the psyche and the soma, and the tension between the scientific method and the patient's needs, the clinician is urged to focus on the process of the practitioner-patient relationship. There is a need to incorporate the insights from George Engel's biopsychosocial model and to develop communication skills that will foster a therapeutic encounter to support the inherent strength of the patient and promote his or her own healing powers.

REFERENCES

1. Barsky, A.J. Hidden reasons some patients visit doctors. *Annals of Internal Medicine,* 1981, *94*(part 1), 492–498.
2. Barrett, J.E., Barrett, J.A., Oxman, T.E., & Gerber, P.D. The prevalence of psychiatric disorders in a primary care practice. *Archives of General Psychiatry,* 1988, *45,* 1100–1106.
3. Norquist, G.S., & Regier, D.A. The epidemiology of psychiatric disorders and the de facto mental health care system. *Annual Review of Medicine,* 1996, *47,* 473–479.
4. Eisenberg, L. Treating depression and anxiety in primary care: Closing the gap between knowledge and practice. *New England Journal of Medicine,* 1992, *326,* 1080–1084.
5. Engel, G.L. The clinical application of the biopsychosocial model. *American Journal of Psychiatry,* 1980, *137,* 535–544.
6. McWhinney, I.R. The meaning of holistic medicine. *Canadian Family Physician,* 1980, *26,* 1097.
7. Dantzer, R. Stress and disease: A psychobiological perspective. *Annuals of Behavioral Medicine,* 1991, *13,* 205–210.
8. Anandarajah, G., & Hight, E. Spirituality and medical practice: Using the HOPE questions as a practical tool for spiritual assessment. *American Family Physician,* 2001, *63*(1), 81–88.
9. Ader, R., Felton, D.L., & Cohen, N. (eds.) *Psychoneuroimmunology,* 2nd ed. San Diego: Academic Press, 1991.
10. Derogatis, C.R., Abeloff, M.D., & Melisaratos, N. Psychological coping mechanisms and survival time in metastatic breast cancer. *Journal of the American Medical Association,* 1979, *242,* 1504–1508.
11. Greer, S., Morris, T., & Pettingale, K.W. Psychological response to breast cancer: Effects on outcome. *Lancet,* 1979, *13,* 785–787.

12. Spiegel, D., Bloom, J., Kraemer, H.C., & Gottheil, E. Effect of psychosocial treatment on the survival of patients with metastatic breast cancer. *Lancet*, 1989, *2*, 888–891.

13. Garsen, B., & Goodkin, K. On the role of immunological factors as mediators between psychosocial factors and cancer progression. *Psychiatry Research*, 1999, *85*, 51–61.

14. Helgeson, V.S., & Cohen, S. Social support and adjustment to cancer: Reconciling descriptive, correlational and intervention research. *Health Psychology*, 1996, *15*, 135–148.

15. Meyer, T.J., & Mark, M.M. Effects of psychosocial interventions with adult cancer patients: A meta-analysis of randomized experiments. *Health Psychology*, 1995, *14*, 101–108.

16. Bartrop, R.W., Lazarus, L., Luckherst, E., Kiloh, L.G., & Penny, R. Depressed lymphocyte function after bereavement. *Lancet*, 1977, *1*, 834–836.

17. Schleifer, S.J., Keller, S.E., Camerino, M., Thornton, J.C., & Stein, M. Suppression of lymphocyte stimulation following bereavement. *Journal of the American Medical Association*, 1983, *250*, 374–377.

18. Cohen, S.C., Tyrrell, D.A.J., & Smith, A.P. Psychological stress and susceptibility to the common cold. *New England Journal of Medicine*, 1991, *325*, 601–611.

19. Kiecolt-Glaser, J.K., & Glaser, R. Mind and immunity. In Goleman, D., & Gurin, J. (eds.) *Mind Body Medicine*. New York: Consumer Reports Books, 1996, pp. 39–61.

20. Weiss, J.M. Behavioral and psychological influences on gastrointestinal pathology: Experimental techniques and findings. In Gentry, W.E. (ed.) *Handbook of Behavioral Medicine*. New York: Guilford Press, 1984, pp. 174–221.

21. Sobel, R.K. The wisdom of the gut. *U.S. News and World Report*, 2000 Apr 3, *128*(3), 50–51.

22. Smith, T.W. Hostility and health: Current status of a psychosomatic hypothesis. *Health Psychology*, 1992, *11*, 139–150.

23. Avery, D., & Winokur, G. Mortality in depressed patients treated with electroconvulsive therapy and antide-pressants. *Archives of General Psychiatry*, 1976, *33*, 1029–1037.

24. Pratt, L.A., Ford, D.E., Crum, R.M., Armenian, H.K., Gallo, J.J., & Eaton, W.W. Depression, psychotropic medication, and risk of myocardial infarction; prospective data from the Baltimore ECA follow-up. *Circulation*, 1996, *94*, 3123–3129.

25. Anda, R., Williamson, D., Jones, D., Macera, C., Eaker, E., Glassman, A., & Marks, J. Depressed affect, hope-lessness, and the risk of ischemic heart disease in a cohort of US adults. *Epidemiology*, 1993, *4*, 285–294.

26. Wassertheil-Smoller, S., Applegate, W.B., Berge, K., Chang, C.J., Davis, B.R., Grimm, R., Jr., Kostis, J., Pressel, S., & Schron, E. Change in depression as a precursor of cardiovascular events. *Archives of Internal Medicine*, 1996, *156*, 553–561.

27. Guck, T.P., Kavan, M.G., Elsasser, G.N., & Barone, E.J. Assessment and treatment of depression following myocardial infarction. *American Family Physician*, 2001, *64*(4), 641–647.

28. Frasure-Smith, N., Lesperance, F., & Talajic, M. Depression following myocardial infarction: Impact on 6-month survival. *Journal of the American Medical Association*, 1993, *270*, 1819–1825.

29. Carney, R.M., Rich, M.W., te Velde, A., Saini, J., Clark, K., & Freedland, K.E. Major depressive disorders in coronary artery disease. *American Journal of Cardiology*, 1987, *60*, 1273–1275.

30. Carney, R.M., Freedland, K.E., & Jaffe, A.S. Insomnia and depression prior to myocardial infarction. *Psychosomatic Medicine*, 1990, *52*, 603–609.

31. Schleifler, S.J., Macari-Hinson, M.M., Coyle, D.A., Slater, W.R., Kahn, M., Gorlin, R., & Zucker, H.D. The nature and course of depression following myocardial infarction. *Archives of Internal Medicine*, 1989, *249*, 1785–1789.

32. Kubzansky, L.D., & Kawachi, I. Going to the heart of the matter: Do negative emotions cause coronary heart disease? *Journal of Psychosomatic Research*, 2000, *48*, 323–337.

33. Tennant, C. Life stress, social support and coronary heart disease. *Australian & New Zealand Journal of Psychiatry*, 1999, *33*, 636–641.

34. Smith, D.F. Negative emotions and coronary heart disease: Causally related or merely coexistent? A review. *Scandinavian Journal of Psychology*, 2001, *42*, 57–69.

35. Lown, B. Introduction. In Cousins, N. *The Healing Heart: Antidotes to Panic and Helplessness*. New York: Norton, 1983, pp. 12–13.

36. Hegetschweiller, K. *New York Times*, April 28, 1998.

37. Astin, J.A. Why patients use alternative medicine. *Journal of the American Medical Association*, 1998, *279*, 1548–1553.

38. Taylor, R.B. Health promotion: Can it succeed in the office? *Preventive Medicine*, 1981, *10*, 258–262.

39. Health Care Financing Administration, Office of the Actuary, 1999.

40. Smith, G.R., Jr., Monson, R.A., & Ray, D.C. Psychiatric consultation in somatization disorder: A randomized controlled study. *New England Journal of Medicine*, 1986, *314*, 1407–1413.

41. Ackerman, A.D., Lyons, J.S., Hammer, J.S., & Larson, D.B. The impact of coexisting depression and timing of psychiatric consultation on medical patients' length of stay. *Hospital and Community Psychiatry*, 1988, *39*, 173–176.

42. Levenson, J.L., Hamer, R.M., & Rossiter, L.F. Relation of psychopathy in general medical inpatients to use and cost of services. *American Journal of Psychiatry*, 1990, *147*, 1498–1503.

43. Frasure-Smith, N. In-hospital symptoms of psychological stress as predictors of long-term outcome after acute myocardial infarction in men. *American Journal of Cardiology*, 1991, *67*, 121–127.

44. Strain, J.J., Lyons, J.S., Hammer, J.S., Fahs, M., Lebovits, A., Paddison, P.L., Synder, S., Strauss, E., Burton, R., Nuber, G., Abernathy, T., Sacks, H., Nordlie, J., & Sacks, C. Cost offset from a psychiatric consultation-liaison intervention with elderly hip fracture patients. *American Journal of Psychiatry*, 1991, *148*, 1044–1049.

45. Guthrie, E., Creed, F., Dawson, D., & Tomenson, B.A. Controlled trial of psychological treatment for the irritable bowel syndrome. *Gastroenterology*, 1991, *100*, 450–457.

46. Starr, P. *The Social Transformation of American Medicine*. New York: Basic Books, 1984, p. 424.

47. Kuhn, T.S. *The Structure of Scientific Revolutions*. Chicago: University of Chicago Press, 1962.

48. Mahoney, M.J. Open exchange and epistemic progress. *American Psychologist*, 1985, *40*, 29.

49. McWhinney, I. *A Textbook of Family Medicine*, 2nd ed. New York: Oxford University Press, 1997, p. 50.

50. Hrobjartsson, A., & Gotzsche, P.C. Is the placebo powerless? *New England Journal of Medicine*, 2001, *344*, 1594–1602.

51. Bailar, J.C. The powerful placebo and the Wizard of Oz. *New England Journal of Medicine*, 2001, *344*, 1630–1632.

52. Frank, J.D. The placebo is psychotherapy. *Behavioral and Brain Sciences*, 1983, *6*, 291–292.

53. Cousins, N. *The Healing Heart: Antidotes to Panic and Helplessness*. New York: Norton, 1983.

54. Engel, G.L. The need for a new medical model: A challenge for biomedicine. *Science*, 1977, *196*, 129–136.

55. McWhinney, I. *Time, Change and the Physician. Plenary Address to the Society of Teachers of Family Medicine*. Sixteenth Annual Spring Conference, Boston, May 1983.

CHAPTER 2

How Patients React to Stress

Neither illness nor health can be understood as purely personal events but must be seen in the context of family and cultural ties. At any given time, the patient and the patient's health are influenced by a multitude of factors, including past experience, the present situation, and expectations for the future.[1]

The Fifteen-Minute Hour outlines simple interventions available to primary care practitioners that will have a major impact on patients' experiences of their illnesses and their lives. The practitioner can minimize the benefit of the "sick role,"[2] foster growth, provide social support, and help both patients and families set realistic expectations for themselves and each other. Considering the social context as part of routine medical treatment enhances the restoration and maintenance of healthier functioning in our patients.

STRESS AND SOCIAL SUPPORT

Our understanding of the stress response as a nonspecific physical reaction comes originally from Hans Selye,[3] who saw stress as a biological mobilization for action, action required to adapt to change. There are many ways to define stress; in fact, stress has been defined not only as a response but also as both cause and even effect of the response.[4] Although the reaction of the autonomic nervous system to perceived danger or demand is often thought of as a standard process (achieving the physiological readiness for fight or flight), many factors mediate the relationship between stress and illness. On an individual or psychological level, these factors include personality traits, coping styles, and the availability of social support. Personality traits, by definition, are set patterns, and coping styles vary in effectiveness, but social support is a resource that can be mobilized rapidly by concerned individuals.

Social support can be understood as a psychological mechanism providing positive information that helps people reassess or redefine perceptions regarding themselves, their situation, or the *quality* of their interpersonal relationships. The information may be about the individual, about the relationship, or about solutions for a problem. It is the positive quality of the social support that aids the individual in developing more positive expectations toward other people and in subsequently behaving in such a manner as to realize these expectations.

Social support appears to have important direct and indirect health effects. Some of the indirect effects of strong social support include healthier coping processes in rheumatoid arthritis patients[5] and greater well-being in breast cancer survivors.[6] Perhaps more compelling are the findings from studies examining the direct effects of social support on health outcomes. For example, maintaining more diverse social networks is associated with greater resistance to the common cold.[7]

Conversely, poor social support appears to be an independent risk factor for acute coronary heart disease events,[8] to interact with life stressors to increase the risk of breast carcinoma,[9] and to predict poor pregnancy outcomes even after the data are controlled for biomedical risk.[10]

Just as every part of the human organism is involved in maintaining homeostasis, each person strives to maintain a personal/social steady state while interfacing with other people. A record of the subjective experience and an interpretation of these interactions with others are stored in people's memories. This recorded information is constantly used to develop expectations for subsequent encounters. It becomes part of a person's "story." The story, and the expectations based on it, continue to affect the person's manner of interacting with others, causing these expectations to become self-fulfilling prophecies. Later chapters will discuss how to listen to and help people modify their stories.

DETERMINING THE CONTEXT OF THE VISIT

Probably the most important question that any practitioner asks about a patient's visit (other than an acute, life-threatening episode) is "Why is the patient coming now?" Mr. Jones has had a sore throat for two weeks. He denies any fever. He has no cough or other symptoms. His throat is slightly erythematous. What made him decide to come today? He does not seem to be that sick. It would seem that he felt at least this bad for the past two weeks. So why did he come in now? The best way to find out what Mr. Jones is concerned about is to ask him: "What are you afraid is going on?" It is also important to get some idea of what is going on in his life. What level of stress is he dealing with? How well are his coping mechanisms working? Does he have adequate social supports? Information about his symptoms in the absence of the context of his current life situation is almost meaningless. The greatest danger lies in getting caught up in the details of Mr. Jones's experience. Many practitioners are reluctant to explore the psychosocial aspects of a patient's problem because of the time-consuming nature of this process. Patients, when encouraged to talk, often consume great amounts of the practitioner's time without coming to any resolution. The practitioner feels battle-weary and behind schedule without the satisfaction of having successfully "treated" anything specific.

Sometimes the practitioner can intervene to reduce the stress, for example, by asking family members to make certain adjustments or by writing an excuse to relieve pressures at work. However, it may be more constructive to suggest ways to modify the perception of the stress or to help the patient develop stress management techniques. In this way, the practitioner helps the patient to moderate the reaction. The stress remains the same. The perception of the stress changes, and the patient reacts differently. *Objectively nothing is changed, but subjectively everything is changed.* A third-year medical student interviewing patients in a local physician's office told the following story:

A 46-year-old woman came into the office complaining of low back pain and bilateral leg pain. She had had this pain for 3 days, and it was getting worse. She said that the pain was constant, was progressive, was "12 on a scale from zero to 10," radiated down both legs, prevented sleep, and was not relieved by anything (she had tried Tylenol, Naprosyn, and Advil). Never in her life had she had this kind of experience. She was in so much pain that she could not eat. She had started to limp that morning. After this full description I asked, "What else is happening in your life?" Her answer was "I'm having troubles at work—the other women working there do not like me." I asked, "How do you feel about that?" She said, "It makes me sad, angry, and terribly frustrated." When I asked, "What troubles you the most?" she answered, "The pain is so bad that I can't work, but I really need this job to survive. I am afraid that I am going to get fired." She paused and then added, "They would really like to see me get fired." I asked, "How are you handling that?" Her reply was "Not very well. I feel totally stressed out." I told her that it sounded like a tough situation to be in and that it must be very hard for her to deal with.

The student paused for effect. Then she added, "I really don't understand what went on there, but when she left the office, she was not limping anymore."

HELPING PATIENTS COPE WITH STRESS RELATED TO THE OFFICE VISIT

An appointment with a practitioner may be stressful for the patient. The first visit can almost be compared to a blind date.[11] Negative past experiences with doctors may cause the patient to anticipate unpleasant experiences and arouse the fight or flight response. Since at this point neither fight nor flight is appropriate, unpleasant body sensations are experienced.

A physical complaint and/or the anxiety attached to a particular problem causes the patient to consult the clinician. The patient may feel anxious in anticipation of having to respond to certain demands, such as requests for personal information or for permission to examine parts of the body—the patient feels physically and emotionally exposed. There is really nothing that a practitioner may not look at, touch, or ask about. There may also be demands to accept the authority of the practitioner, to please him or her, to follow instructions, to be a "good" patient. The patient may feel stressed in the dependent role and out of control in this situation. An illustration of this response is provided by recent studies of the white-coat hypertension response that have consistently shown that approximately 40% of patients have systolic or diastolic blood pressure readings in the office setting at least 10 points higher than readings taken at home.[12-14]

The Medical Appointment as a Source of Stress

The sources of stress related to the office visit can be divided into three basic categories. Almost all patients come to doctors because of *pain or anxiety about a symptom or illness* and thus experience a basic level of stress right from the start. The second category of stress has to do with *logistics*. The patient must make an appointment, take time off from work, get transportation, arrive and wait in the examining room, fill out countless forms, and provide payment. The third category concerns the *interpersonal elements* of the visit. Patients may feel stressed as they anticipate questions, judgments, scoldings, praise, instructions, and ultimately the diagnosis that the practitioner will pronounce. There are certain "demand characteristics"[15] that have to do with being a "good patient." Some of this is learned behavior on the part of the patient. This learning is greatly influenced by family or cultural perceptions of the "patient's role." Since the practitioner's expectations regarding the patient's behavior and the patient's expectations regarding the practitioner's behavior may not always coincide, more stress can be created.

Minimizing the Patient's Stress

By recognizing the effect of the situation on the patient's behavior, the practitioner can help to relieve much stress or anxiety experienced by the patient. A classic article in the *Journal of the American Medical Association* cited the effectiveness of empathic understanding in calming anxious patients.[16] Practitioners can use key phrases to address the patient's response to a stressful situation, to make it overt, and to legitimize or normalize it. As we have said earlier, just recognizing a situation as a problem changes it. By acknowledging, "It must be difficult for you to get here in the middle of your busy day," or, "You have had to wait a long time and must be quite impatient," the practitioner provides support and helps the patient to relax.

In the real world of everyday practice, unfortunately, even if practitioners address the issue of patient convenience, instead of focusing on the patient's experience and providing empathy, they generally explain why they were detained and cite numerous emergencies or situations involving other patients with more acute needs. This underscores the practitioner's importance and minimizes the patient's significance. The resulting decreased level of self-esteem makes it more difficult for the patient to cope, thereby increasing stress. These concepts will be discussed further in subsequent chapters.

When we acknowledge that the patient has a right to be annoyed or upset by having to wait and that this is a reasonable response to the situation, we have given support. One element of support is approval, or at least acceptance, of a person's behavior. In giving support, we provide relief. Our aim is always to alleviate the patient's psychological distress. We prefer to recognize and accept reactions rather than explain them. As Fritz Perls[17] has emphatically stated, the *what* and *how* are important, not the *why*. It may make little sense to us that patients feel a particular way. However, rather than trying to talk patients out of how they feel or figuring out why they feel that way, we acknowledge those feelings and deal with them in a practical, therapeutic, time-effective way.

Many issues determine the patient's expectations in the doctor-patient relationship. These issues include patients' illness stories,[18,19] their requests,[20] and various explanatory models of illness growing out of the patient's cultural heritage.[2,21] Full discussion of these elements is beyond the scope of this book. However, when patients exhibit anxiety, whether related to the stress of a comprehensive examination, potential diagnosis, or other life stress, it is most important *not* to say, "You have no reason to feel anxious!" If the patient actually had no reason to feel anxious, the patient would not feel that way. Instead, we recommend saying, "I can understand that you would feel anxious in this situation. Let's see what we can do to make you feel better."

WHY PATIENTS ADAPT DIFFERENTLY TO STRESS

When mental health is poor, individuals are more likely to develop disease and are much less tolerant of physical symptoms.[22,23] The correlation between illness and stressful life events is generally accepted. In 1951, Holmes, Treuting, and Wolff[24] first documented the effects of life situations and the accompanying emotional reactions on patients with hay fever. Holmes and Rahe[25] went on to standardize their schedule of recent life events that has been widely used in research. However, many people under stress do not develop disease. These people seem to resist diseases developed by others and seem to prosper both physically and mentally, even under traumatic conditions. What makes them so different?

The "Salutogenic" Model

Aaron Antonovsky[26,27] has studied the factors that seem to protect people from the consequences of stress. He suggests that when we are studying people's reactions to stress it is useful to switch from a pathogenic to a "salutogenic" model. In explaining why some people stay healthy regardless of what happens to them, Antonovsky first specifies what he calls generalized resistance resources, such as constitutionally good health, knowledge and intelligence, education, access to money, and a rational, flexible, and far-sighted coping style. He suggests that given a sufficient amount of quality generalized resistance resources in childhood and adolescence, the individual will develop what Antonovsky calls a "sense of coherence." This characteristic seems to insulate a person from having negative health consequences, even from stressful events that cause disease in people who are more vulnerable. The sense of coherence is basically a stable psychological orientation in which individuals are able to make sense out of different aspects of their lives, weaving their experience into a coherent whole. They are able to put the pieces of their lives together and maintain a basic faith that, generally, "things will work out as well as can reasonably be expected," which they consider to be all right. A strong sense of coherence has been shown to predict good health in both men and women.[28] In clinical practice, this sense of coherence is an important concept that can be applied therapeutically, as discussed later.

To be able to connect aspects of our experience into a coherent whole is important, as is connecting to other people. It is the loss of the sense of being connected that seems to be a critical factor in feeling and becoming vulnerable. Cassel[29] first described this phenomenon and suggested that the subjective interpretation, or personal experience, of an ill person induces a loss of connectedness. It is interesting to note that Kobasa's original concept of hardiness[30] specified qualities of commitment, challenge, control, and connection. Hardiness distinguishes people who do not develop illness under stress. Hardy personalities find some way to make a meaningful commitment to the task, retain a sense of perceived control by focusing on their own behavior, redefine situations as a challenge, and connect with other people in supportive ways. Based on *hardiness* scores, Kobasa, Maddi, and Courington[31] were able to predict differences in illness response among executives stressed by similar life changes. It is the sensed loss of control that may make a person vulnerable, by compromising the immune system. Epidemiological evidence is accumulating that psychological distress may play a causal role in both morbidity and mortality.[32,33]

A LOOK AT THE DATA

Let us look at several sets of research findings. First, we will examine a prospective, longitudinal study that relates mental and physical health.[22,23,34,35] Next, we will discuss both theoretical and empirical data that indicate that every person has at least two levels of functioning. Finally, we will show how functioning under stress relates to the person's locus of control.[36]

A Longitudinal Study of Adaptation

In his book *Adaptation to Life*,[34] George Vaillant details the lives of a large number of the subjects of the Grant Study of Adult Development, a comprehensive prospective study that has so far observed 237 initially healthy college men for 55 years. Initial data were collected through repeated physical examinations and by interviews and comprehensive questionnaires for the longitudinal monitoring of psychological, social, and occupational adjustments. All important life events were observed. Among other characteristics carefully studied were the types of symptoms that the subjects developed under stress. This research clearly demonstrated the connection between healthy psychological functioning and healthy physical functioning. Further, after carefully analyzing his data, Vaillant concluded that there was little evidence to support the existence of specific mental diseases, only evidence of maladaptive reactions to stress.

Vaillant found that people change over time, generally "maturing" psychologically as they grow older. He also found that some people are healthier than others. Under favorable circumstances, mental health develops and is correlated with robust physical health. This also generally predisposes the person to success in the work environment. Both physical health and mental health depend on successful adaptation. In a later report published in the *New England Journal of Medicine*,[22] Vaillant reported that poor physical health accompanied and was followed by poor mental health. Conversely, poor mental health (i.e., poor adaptation to stressful life events) was a clear predictor of subsequent poor physical health. In a follow-up after 45 years of the study,[35] psychosocial factors gathered before age 50 years were examined in relation to physical health, mental health, and life satisfaction at age 65 years. It is interesting that the extent of tranquilizer use before 50 years (hardly the best response to managing stress) was the most powerful negative predictor of both physical and mental health. Paradoxically, a warm, supportive childhood environment made an important independent contribution to predicting *physical* health.[35] In the most recent follow-up after 55 years of the study, Vaillant reported that a group of 64 men who had never used mood-altering drugs or consulted a psychiatrist before the age of 50 years had significantly better health and lower mortality at age 70 years than the rest of the group.[22] Vaillant also concluded that the risk of a mood disorder lies on a continuum from lifelong resistance to vulnerability.

Successful Adaptation Defines Health

Vaillant found that individual traumatic incidents did not generally have dramatic effects on the quality of people's lives. Rather, people's lives, in general, seemed to have a relatively stable course.[34] It was successfully adapting to problems, not the absence of stressors, that determined healthy functioning and growth. Vaillant determined a range of adaptive (defense) mechanisms. He proposed four lines of defenses: psychotic, immature, neurotic, and mature.

Defense mechanisms such as delusional projection, denial, and distortion, which are part of the psychotic level, are normal for individuals under the age of five years. Immature mechanisms, such as projection, hypochondriases, and acting out, are common in healthy three- to fifteen-year-olds. The neurotic defenses outlined by Vaillant are intellectualization, repression, and reaction formation, which are commonly seen in "healthy individuals ages three to ninety, in neurotic disorder, and in mastering acute adult stress."[37] Mature mechanisms, such as altruism, humor, suppression, anticipation, and sublimation, are normal in healthy individuals of all ages. Under stress, however, they may change to less mature mechanisms. When demands from the internal or external environments become too great for the mature defense mechanisms to handle, the individual temporarily makes a retreat to more primitive defenses. This may be labeled "regressing," or under severe conditions it is seen as "decompensating."

Extreme stress causes individuals to regress from their characteristic coping mechanisms to poorer or less mature ones. These more primitive coping mechanisms provide less successful adaptation and therefore potentiate poorer mental and physical health. The most important finding according to Vaillant[34] is not that stress kills us but that ingenious adaptation to stress, which he calls "good mental health," facilitates our survival. Vaillant's work provides support for the themes that are central to this text:

1. Mental health and physical health are inextricably linked.
2. Individuals use different coping mechanisms under stress than when not under stress.
3. In general, individuals have consistent coping patterns. They use specific patterns at a particular level of maturity under normal circumstances and less functional patterns under stress.
4. It is most important to support people under stress in order to help them return to more adaptive defenses.

A Holistic Theory of Neurosis

Vaillant comes from a psychoanalytical school of psychiatry. A psychiatrist with a very different orientation, who provides interesting theoretical support for the conclusions of the Grant study, is discussed below.

Andras Angyal's work is not well known in the medical community. Angyal[38] was a successful analyst who proposed a theory and treatment of neurosis that he labeled a "holistic method." His theory is useful because it provides a plausible explanation for the uncomfortable phenomena that people experience when they are under overwhelming stress. Angyal also provides direction for producing relief.

Angyal's theory of human nature and personality posits that two systems, one healthy and one neurotic, vie for dominance in our personality. All persons have a need to feel competent, or, as Angyal puts it, there is a drive for autonomy. There is also a companion need to belong, which Angyal calls the need for homonomy, essentially a feeling of connectedness. The healthy system develops through the experience of having one's basic needs met, that is, both feeling personally competent and also feeling accepted by significant others in one's life. The healthy system is based on feeling both loved (connected) and effective as an autonomous person (competent). The world of the healthy personality is a reasonably safe and loving place. Conversely, the neurotic system builds on experiences of feeling incompetent, rejected, or resentful. It registers only needs that have been unfulfilled. Angyal suggests that since no life, however unfortunate, is all trauma, the basic data processed by the two systems are actually the same. Angyal says that we actually live in two worlds. Both are complete systems, and they vie for dominance. We never live in the world proper, but we create our map of the world,[39] which is not the same as the territory.[40] Moreover, Angyal tells us that we actually have two different maps, which we use under different circumstances.

We relate to the world either with reasonably positive expectations using our healthy map or with unreasonable fear and discomfort using our neurotic map. When the neurotic system is engaged, the world seems hostile, threatening, and withholding, and our primary aim is to protect ourselves and escape danger. The world feels huge and menacing while we feel small and inadequate. This belief system prevents us from feeling safe or optimistic. Danger exists everywhere. Until our healthy self has been reengaged, we cannot feel hope or problem solve confidently.

Support helps to restore people's sense of trust in the world that is represented by the healthy personality system. Therapeutic interventions by the practitioner that cause the patient to feel competent and connected will reengage the healthy system.

Research From Experimental Psychology

Although shaped in different language, physiological experimental psychology has demonstrated specific responses in subjects under stress. As people become overaroused (tense and overstimulated), they filter out parts of current experience: coping mechanisms become more primitive in several ways, including reversion to more dominant, first-learned behaviors. When recently learned behavior is not available, those responses that might be most appropriate to the situation are temporarily blocked and cannot be utilized. Novel stimuli are not recognized. Under highly aroused conditions, people revert to "overlearned" responses. This means they automatically use behavior that has been done so often that it requires no conscious thought.[41] When levels of arousal are brought back to a comfortable level, problem solving becomes effective again. Recently learned material returns as part of the behavioral repertoire, increasing the variety of options available. Mental health is restored.

Therapeutic Implications

The connecting thread among these viewpoints confirms our personal clinical experience that facing unmanageable stressors puts people on *tilt*. For many people there are degrees of diminishing functioning under stress, perhaps even a peak of efficiency before the decline sets in, but there appears to be a threshold that precipitates behavior characteristic of overstressed (overaroused) functioning for each individual. Having passed this threshold, people click in their neurotic map of the world and then act as though that is the only reality they know. For the practitioner, the primary therapeutic task is to provide support in order to restore people's equilibrium and refocus them in their healthier orientation. This is often not difficult. K.E. Weik has pointed out that simply labeling a problem as minor rather than serious lowers people's arousal level. He suggested that this is particularly beneficial when "people don't know what to do or are unable to do it."[42] Often practitioners can point out that there is a difference between problems that are urgent and those that are important. More will be said about this in later chapters.

Internal or External Locus of Control

Locus of control[36] is a critical concept in understanding people's reactions to stressful circumstances and designing appropriate interventions. Whether the person is feeling healthy, safe, and in control or neurotic, unsafe, and out of control, the feeling of safety, or lack thereof, is a purely subjective one that is affected by the person's locus of control. Locus of control is an important construct that few practitioners consciously apply. People's health-related behavior is strongly influenced by their locus of control.[43,44] Individuals with an internal locus of control cope best when they have the resources (information, power, time) to handle a situation, whereas individuals with an external locus of control feel safe when a trusted authority figure has taken charge and told them what to do or when family or community resources have been recruited for their support. The implications for medical practice and for dealing with patients and others under stress are obvious.

The practitioner who understands the issues involved in these three areas of research—the relationship between psychological and physical well-being, the regression to more primitive functioning whenever defenses are overwhelmed, and security based on internal or external locus of control—will be able to make effective interventions, at critical times, with little investment of time, energy, or effort.

APPLICATION TO ILLNESS BEHAVIOR

The effects of acute illness constitute a high degree of stress. People's behavior under these circumstances can be better understood by reviewing the normal developmental process by which human beings mature. Chris Argyris, writing from the point of view of organizational psychology, specified five dimensions of individual development.[45] As people mature, they move along a continuum from being passive to being active; from dependence to independence; from requiring immediate gratification of their needs to being able to delay gratification for long periods; from concrete thinking to abstract thinking; and from having few abilities to having many abilities. At any given time, each person functions at a specific level on each of these dimensions. The more highly developed or mature the individual, the higher the level of functioning along each axis that can be expected. In circumstances of acute stress, people will temporarily regress along each of the five dimensions, although not necessarily to the same extent. Vaillant's findings confirmed these phenomena.

Acute illness is an acute stress. There is an acute regression of functioning. People who are ill become more passive and more dependent, want their demands met instantly, become more concrete in their thinking, and have fewer abilities to help themselves. This can try the patience of the caregiver but can be more easily handled if it is anticipated and perceived to be transitory. In chronic illness, unfortunately, the regression often becomes permanent. Practitioners aware of this dynamic can prevent further stress by helping caregivers to set realistic expectations for the patient and the course of the illness while providing support to maximize return to premorbid levels of functioning.

Results of Being Overwhelmed

The subjective feeling of being overwhelmed contributes to the objective inability of individuals to function at optimum levels. The resulting perception of inadequacy lowers the individual's sense of self-esteem. These feelings can be transient, lasting only several seconds, or they may constitute the general phenomenological experience of the individual. Often negative experiences of the self are specific to particular, symbolically threatening situations. At other times, they may be precipitated and maintained by traumatic life events or by an accumulation of daily hassles.[6] No particular situation or event is considered to be inherently stressful; rather, it is the individual's interpretation of the situation as threatening or harmful that defines it as a stressor.[46] William James[47] first suggested that emotions and their effects on our bodies are objective phenomena that are determined through the subjective experience:

> Our natural way of thinking about these . . . emotions is that the mental perception of some fact excites the mental affection called the emotion, and that this latter state of mind gives rise to the bodily expression. My theory on the contrary, is that the bodily changes follow directly on the perception of the exciting fact, and that our feeling of the same changes as they occur IS the emotion. Common sense says, we lose our fortune, are sorry and weep; we meet a bear, are frightened and run; we are insulted by a rival, are angry and strike. The hypothesis here to be defended says that this order of sequence is incorrect, that the one mental state is not immediately induced by the other, that the bodily manifestations must first be interposed between, and that the more rational statement is that we feel sorry because we cry, angry because we strike, or tremble because we are sorry, angry, or fearful, as the case may be. Without the bodily states following on the perception, the latter would be purely cognitive in form, pale, colorless, destitute of emotional warmth. We might then see the bear, and judge it best to run, receive the insult and deem it right to strike, but we should not actually feel afraid or angry.

When we feel basically in control of our responses to the events happening in our lives (appropriately able to flee, fight, or flow), we function at an effective level. As long as the demands of the external environment (other people) and internal environment (expectations for the self) are experienced as manageable, we will continue to function at our customary level. Once the tolerance for comfortable adaptation has been exceeded, however, we begin to use a different coping style. At the extreme, Martin Seligman has shown that once people are convinced that events are completely beyond their control and that their behavior will in no way affect the outcome of a particular situation, they behave in a stereotyped manner that he has labeled "learned helplessness."[48] This is an emotional sequence that involves going through a fear-protest stage to a helpless-depressed stage. The more out of control the person feels, the more primitive are the defenses called into play. Although this response appears to be ineffective, it is a person's best effort to survive when in an overwhelmed state.

Each of us can usually identify when we are feeling overwhelmed by observing our behavior. We go on *tilt* and are momentarily unable to do anything about it. Sometimes our awareness can help us engage strategies to restore our equilibrium. In many cases, however, our perception of our behavior, and our inability to control or modify it, exacerbates the feelings of being overwhelmed. When we lose faith in our power to manage at all, we fall into our dependent mode and look to be taken care of. When there is no one to do this or when we do not trust the person who is in charge, we become despondent and helpless.

Research has shown that over time this type of stress can contribute to a compromise of the defense systems of the body and lead to subsequent disease.[49-52] At first, patients are simply aware of symptoms, such as muscle tension, which may be experienced as back, neck, or head pain. Patients may become aware of a rapid pulse, abdominal pain, breathing difficulties, blurred vision, a full bladder, diarrhea, sweating, a tight throat, or difficulty swallowing. Other, less noticeable body reactions triggered by the sympathetic nervous system–mediated stress-response syndrome may result in elevated blood pressure, elevated lipid levels, changes in blood sugar, suppression of the immune system, and ultimately the compromise of various organ systems.[53]

THE CRISIS INTERVENTION MODEL

A crisis may be thought of as an environmentally produced situation to which the individual must respond, such as a disaster, an accident, the loss of a job, or the death of a loved one. There are also normal developmental crises (also called transition points) in the life cycle. A crisis may be thought of most simply as the time of greatest change or potential change. Practitioners generally define a crisis as a clinical syndrome, involving emotional upset, increased tension, unpleasant affect, breakdown of coping mechanisms, and disorganized functioning. A situation is experienced as a crisis when an individual perceives an event as threatening to the self in some highly significant way. It is a time of acute stress. People present in crisis, but they come in complaining of organic problems. The first step is to identify the precipitant and then to seize the opportunity to be therapeutic. Crisis is a time when certain decisions have to be made because the previous *status quo* no longer exists, and some adaptive behavior is required. These are important decisions that will affect the subsequent options available. However, crisis is also a time when because of the emotional overlay, the individual is least capable of thinking clearly or problem solving effectively.

George Caplan,[54] explaining the effectiveness of crisis intervention, suggests that each person generally functions within a specific range of effectiveness and personal satisfaction. We have seen this empirically demonstrated by Vaillant.[22,23,34] There is a continuum of functioning, from people who are generally very ineffective to those who are well adjusted and adapted and who enjoy living. In general, people are quite static in their level of functioning, regularly fluctuating within a given range as they experience manageable life stress. As stated previously, in a crisis there is an overwhelming amount of emotional distress preventing the individual from being able to process information objectively or solve problems effectively. Since a crisis is defined as the time of greatest change, regardless of the nature or degree of adaptation required, crisis by definition is time limited.[54] Some resolution will occur within a time span of four to six weeks. The distressed individual is generally eager to receive help, having temporarily moved down on the dependency scale. This affords the practitioner an opportunity to intervene effectively at a time when the individual is open and highly suggestible.

The Goal of Crisis Intervention

Crisis intervention aims to achieve very specific and limited outcomes. There are four general objectives. The first is to prevent dire consequences. In a crisis, the individual is forced to deal with new situations at a time when the ability to solve problems is compromised. The intervening person can suggest that no decision be made that is not absolutely crucial and that those issues that must be resolved be talked through carefully with a disinterested person.

The second objective is to return the individual to the premorbid level of functioning. As discussed previously, providing support that makes the person feel competent and connected will help to achieve this outcome.

Expanding the behavioral repertoire and enhancing self-esteem are the two other objectives of crisis intervention. Weathering the crisis and finding new ways to manage problems and negotiate personal relationships not only expand the behavioral repertoire but also create a positive change in self-esteem and the sense of self-efficacy.

We encourage practitioners to provide symptom relief along with empathy for the subjective experiences of distress. In addition, the clinician can function in the supportive role by providing information and explanations, exploring options, or simply pointing out that options exist and prescribing "tincture of time." Most of all, the practitioner can encourage new behavior that will help the patient to manage the crisis and attain a better level of functioning when psychological equilibrium and physical equilibrium are restored.

Expected Outcomes

If the resolution of the crisis is favorable, the individual can be expected to function at a higher level of adjustment. New coping skills are learned, and confidence in self and others is enhanced. Conversely, if no help is available or if the individual is unable to solve the problem successfully, with or without help, because by definition crises are time limited, the situation will still be resolved but at the cost of a subsequent lower level of functioning. People will move down the scale in all five of Argyris's dimensions.[45]

As we have suggested, during a time of crisis an individual experiences increased dependency needs, wishes to be helped, and signals this to the environment. One of the most efficient ways of signaling for help in our society is to develop an illness, either an acute illness or the exacerbation of a chronic condition. The visit to the practitioner is a cry for help and for symptom relief. It affords the aware practitioner a unique opportunity to invest a few minutes making a therapeutic intervention that has the potential to provide both short-term and long-term benefits for the patient.

APPLICATION TO THE OFFICE SETTING

Some patients at first seem reluctant to discuss their psychological condition when they seek medical treatment. The following example is quite typical of our practice:

Mrs. Z is a 53-year-old schoolteacher who has come to the office for the second time. Her presenting complaint is a sinus problem; she reports having had congestion and severe recurrent headaches for the past three days. Mrs. Z has a history of chronic sinusitis, but this time she says the symptoms have persisted for a longer time than usual. Mrs. Z is a well-dressed, reserved white female who appears somewhat anxious to get out of the office. When she is asked about her current life situation, she reluctantly admits that she is working two jobs and is separated from her husband, but she states that everything is under control. She refuses to give any details of her current situation, and when asked how she feels about her separation she denies that she has any problems and says that she does not want to talk about it. Physical examination is normal. The practitioner then explains to her that sometimes stress and emotional problems have a way of lowering the body resistance and making physical symptoms persist longer or be more difficult to treat. If these problems are not recognized and dealt with, physical health is compromised. The practitioner just presents this explanation to help the patient make sense out of both her current situation and her reaction to it. Deciding to give the patient a few minutes to think about it, he then leaves the room to get a prescription pad. When he returns, he notes that the patient is looking much more relaxed. She says, "Doctor, I really didn't mind you asking me questions about my separation and so forth. It was good that you did. I really have to start dealing with all that stuff." The doctor then schedules her for an appointment the following week, primarily to talk about her psychosocial situation. She leaves feeling much better.

We have tried to show that the practitioner usually sees patients at a time when they are feeling vulnerable. Interventions at this time are very effective, both in restoring the patient's equilibrium and in promoting constructive change. The therapeutic goal is always to make the patient feel both competent and connected. Specific techniques and detailed rationales will be discussed in subsequent chapters. The practitioner is in a unique position to help the patient at an opportune time and is equipped with a variety of valuable skills, as discussed in Chapter 3.

SUMMARY

The stress response is a biologically programmed mobilization for adaptive action in response to changes in the external or internal environments. The visit to the practitioner is usually triggered by distress felt in response to situational factors. Patients also experience stress in regard to the office visit and their interaction with the practitioner. This can be reduced through specific strategies.

In general, there is a relationship between illness and adaptation to life events. Good mental health potentiates physical well-being. Some people are characteristically healthier than others. Drawing from a variety of sources, we present two central concepts: first, that individuals generally function at a specific level of adaptation and, second, that individuals under severe stress, including physical illness, temporarily regress to lower levels of functioning. People with an internal locus of control primarily need to feel competent and in control, whereas people with an external locus of control primarily need to feel connected to a trusted caretaker.

When individuals are in a state of being overwhelmed, they are unable to function at optimum levels. They go on *tilt* and engage their neurotic map of the world. Social support, which provides information regarding an individual's basic acceptability and competence, is crucial at this time.

We relate to the world either with positive expectations, using our healthy map, or with fear and discomfort, using our neurotic map. When the neurotic system is engaged, the world seems threatening, hostile, and withholding, and our main aim is to protect ourselves and escape danger. We feel as though the world is too large and we are too small and inadequate. When caught up in our neurosis, we feel angry, anxious, and isolated. This belief system makes it impossible to feel safe or optimistic. Danger is to be found everywhere. Until our healthy self is reengaged, we cannot feel hope or confidence. The role of the supportive person is to restore the sense of trust in the world that is represented by the healthy personality system. When the actions of the practitioner make the patient feel competent and connected, the healthy system will be reengaged.

The crisis intervention model is useful in specifying the time-limited nature of acute stress. Crises generally resolve within four to six weeks. By providing support, crisis intervention aims to prevent dire consequences, return the individual to a premorbid level of functioning, enhance self-esteem, and expand subsequent coping abilities. If practitioners understand these mechanisms and routinely provide supportive interventions, the results will be therapeutic for patients and rewarding for the practitioner.

REFERENCES

1. McWhinney, I.R. Beyond diagnosis: An approach to the integration of behavioral science and clinical medicine. *New England Journal of Medicine*, 1972, *287*, 384–387.
2. Kleinman, A., Eisenberg, L., & Good, B. Clinical lessons from anthropologic and cross-cultural research. *Annals of Internal Medicine*, 1978, *88*, 251–258.
3. Selye, H. *The Stress of Life*. New York: McGraw-Hill, 1957.
4. Selye, H. The evolution of the stress concept. *American Scientist*, 1973, *61*, 692–699.

5. Griffen, K.W., Friend, R., Kaell, A.T., & Bennett, R.S. Distress and disease status among patients with rheumatoid arthritis: Roles of coping styles and perceived responses from support providers. *Annals of Behavioral Medicine*, 2001, *23*, 133–138.

6. Dirksen, S.R. Predicting well-being among breast cancer survivors. *Journal of Advanced Nursing*, 2000, *32*, 937–943.

7. Cohen, S., Doyle, W.J., Skoner, D.P., Rabin, B.S., & Gwaltney, J.M., Jr. Social ties and susceptibility to the common cold. *Journal of the American Medical Association*, 1997, *277*(24), 1940–1944.

8. Tennant, C. Life stress, social support and coronary heart disease. *Australian & New Zealand Journal of Psychiatry*, 1999, *33*, 636–641.

9. Price, M.A., Tennant, C.C., Butow, P.N., Smith, R.C., Kennedy, S.J., Kossoff, M.B., & Dunn, S.M. The role of psychosocial factors in the development of breast carcinoma. II. Life event stressors, social support, defense style, and emotional control and their interactions. *Cancer*, 2001, *91*, 686–697.

10. Feldman, P.J., Dunkel-Schetter, C., Sandman, C.A., & Wadhwa, P.D. Maternal social support predicts birth weight and fetal growth in human pregnancy. *Psychosomatic Medicine*, 2000, *62*, 715–725.

11. Robinson, S., & Lieberman, J.A. Reducing new patients' anxiety during the first visit. *Family Practice Management*, 1998, *5*, 54–61.

12. Lerman, C.E., Brody, D.S., Hui, T., Lazaro, C., Smith, D.G., & Blum, M.J. The white-coat hypertension response: Prevalence and predictors. *Journal of General Internal Medicine*, 1989, *4*, 226–231.

13. White, W.B., Schulman, P., & McCabe, E.J. Average daily blood pressure, not office blood pressure, determines cardiac function in patients with hypertension. *Journal of the American Medical Association*, 1989, *261*, 873–877.

14. MacDonald, M.B., Laing, G.P., Wilson, M.P., & Wilson, T.W. Prevalence and predictors of the white coat response in patients with treated hypertension. *Canadian Medical Association Journal*, 1999, *161*(3), 265–269.

15. Orne, M.T. On the social demand characteristics and their implications. *American Psychologist*, 1962, *17*, 776–783.

16. Bellet, P.S., & Maloney, M.J. The importance of empathy as an interviewing skill in medicine. *Journal of the American Medical Association*, 1991, *266*, 1831–1832.

17. Perls, F.S. *Gestalt Therapy Verbatim.* Moab, Utah: Real People Press, 1969.

18. Brody, H. *Stories of Sickness.* New Haven, Conn.: Yale University Press, 1987.

19. Kleinman, A. *The Illness Narratives.* New York: Basic Books, 1988.

20. Mechanic, D. Response factors in illness: The studies of illness behavior. In Jaco, G. (ed.) *Patients, Practitioners, Illness: A Source Book in Behavioral Science and Health.* New York: The Free Press, 1979.

21. Lazare, A., & Eisenthal, S. A negotiated approach to the clinical encounter. I. Attending the patient's perspective. In Lazare, A. (ed.) *Outpatient Psychiatry.* Baltimore: Williams & Wilkins, 1979, pp. 157–171.

22. Vaillant, G.E. Natural history of male psychologic health: Effects of mental health on physical health. *New England Journal of Medicine*, 1979, *301*, 1249–1254.

23. Vaillant, G.E., & Gerber, P.D. Natural history of male psychological health. XIV. Relationship of mood disorder vulnerability to physical health. *American Journal of Psychiatry*, 1998, *155*, 184–191.

24. Holmes, T.H., Treuting, T., & Wolff, H.G. Life situations, emotions and nasal disease: Evidence on summative effects exhibited in patients with "hay fever." *Psychosomatic Medicine*, 1951, *13*, 71–82.

25. Holmes, T.H., & Rahe, R.H. The social readjustment rating scale. *Psychosomatic Medicine*, 1967, *11*, 213–218.

26. Antonovsky, A. *Health, Stress, and Coping.* San Francisco: Jossey-Bass, 1979.

27. Antonovsky, A. *Unraveling the Mystery of Health: How People Manage Stress and Stay Well.* San Francisco: Jossey-Bass, 1987.

28. Suominen, S., Helenius, H., Blomberg, H., Uutela, A., & Koskenvuo, M. Sense of coherence as a predictor of subjective state of health: Results of 4 years of follow-up of adults. *Journal of Psychosomatic Research*, 2001, *50*, 77–86.

29. Cassel, J. The contribution of the social environment to host resistance. *American Journal of Epidemiology*, 1976, *104*, 107–123.

30. Kobasa, S.C. Stressful life events, personality, and health: An inquiry into hardiness. *Journal of Personality and Social Psychology*, 1979, *37*, 1–11.

31. Kobasa, S.C., Maddi, S.R., & Courington, S. Personality and constitution as mediators in the stress-illness relationship. *Journal of Health and Social Behavior*, 1981, 368–378.

32. Somervell, P.D., Kaplan, B.H., Heiss, G., Tyroler, H.A., Kleinbaum, D.G., & Obrist, P.A. Psychologic distress as a predictor of mortality. *American Journal of Epidemiology*, 1989, *130*, 1013–1023.

33. Williams, R., Kiecolt-Glaser, J., Legato, M.J., Ornish, D., Powell, L.H., Syme, S.L., & Williams, V. The impact of emotions on cardiovascular health. *Journal of Gender Specific Medicine*, 1999, 2(5), 52–58.

34. Vaillant, G.E. *Adaptation to Life*. Boston: Little, Brown & Co., 1977.

35. Vaillant, G.E., & Vaillant, C.O. Natural history of male psychological health. XII. A 45-year study of predictors of successful aging at age 65. *American Journal of Psychiatry*, 1990, *147*, 31–37.

36. Rotter, J.B. Generalized expectancies for internal versus external control of reinforcement. *Psychological Monographs*, 1966, *80*(l, Whole No. 609).

37. Vaillant. *Adaptation to Life*, p. 384.

38. Angyal, A. *Neurosis and Treatment: A Holistic Theory*. New York: John Wiley & Sons, 1965.

39. Korzybski, A. *Science & Sanity*, 4th ed. Lakeville, Conn.: The International Non-Aristotelian Library Publishing Co., 1958.

40. Bateson, G. *Mind and Nature: A Necessary Unity*. New York: E.P. Dutton, 1979.

41. Staw, B.M., Sandelands, L.E., & Dutton, J.E. Threat-rigidity effects in organizational behavior: A multilevel analysis. *Administrative Science Quarterly*, 1981, *26*, 501–524.

42. Weik, K.E. Small wins: Redefining the scale of social problems. *American Psychologist*, 1984, *39*, 41.

43. Wallston, B.S., Wallston, K.A., Kaplan, G.D., & Maides, S.A. Development and validation of the health locus of control (HCL) scale. *Journal of Consulting and Clinical Psychology*, 1976, *44*, 580–585.

44. Janz, N.K., & Becker, M.H. The health belief model: A decade later. *Health Education Quarterly*, 1984, *11*, 1–47.

45. Argyris, C. *Intervention Theory and Method: A Behavioral Science View*. Reading, Mass.: Addison-Wesley, 1970.

46. Zakowski, S.G., Hall, M.H., Klein, L.C., & Baum, A. Appraised control, coping and stress in a community sample: A test of the goodness-of-fit hypothesis. *Annals of Behavioral Medicine*, 2001, *23*(3), 158–165.

47. James, W. *The Principles of Psychology*, vol. 2. New York: Holt, 1913, pp. 449–450.

48. Seligman, M.E.P. *Helplessness: On Depression, Development, and Death*. San Francisco: Freeman, 1975.

49. Christie-Seely, J. Life stress and illness: A systems approach. *Canadian Family Physician*, 1983, *29*, 533–540.

50. Watson, D., & Pennebaker, J.W. Health complaints, stress and distress: Exploring the central role of negative affectivity. *Psychological Review*, 1989, *96*, 234–254.

51. Glaser, R., Rabin, B., Chesney, M., Cohen, S., & Natelson, B. Stress-induced immunomodulation: Implications for infectious diseases? *Journal of the American Medical Association*, 1999, *281*, 2268–2270.

52. Mayne, T.J., Vittinghoff, E., Chesney, M.A., Barrett, D.C., & Coates, T.J. Depressive affect and survival among gay and bisexual men infected with HIV. *Archives of Internal Medicine*, 1996, *156*, 2233–2238.

53. Maier, S.F., & Watkins, L.R. Cytokines for psychologists: Implications of bidirectional immune-to-brain communication for understanding behavior, mood and cognition. *Psychological Review*, 1998, *105*(1), 83–107.

54. Caplan, G. *Principles of Preventive Psychiatry*. New York: Basic Books, 1964.

CHAPTER 3

The Psychotherapeutic Qualifications of the Primary Care Practitioner

Since emotional problems often manifest as physical problems and physical problems usually have emotional consequences, physical and emotional problems must be addressed in an integrated manner. Adequate primary care medical treatment is really not possible without confronting the psychosocial dimension. Whether or not the practitioner invites or even desires it, patients often expect help with emotional problems along with physical problems. The practitioner becomes a therapist by default.

THE REALITY OF BEING ON THE SPOT

Are primary care practitioners really qualified and competent to handle emotional problems? The good news is that patients think they are. An impressive literature shows that patients clearly consider these clinicians to be their primary source of mental healthcare.[1,2] A comprehensive study found that patients with psychosocial problems confided in their primary care practitioner more often than any other type of professional. The types of problems included depression, anxiety, bereavement, marital conflicts, problems with children, and other practical problems, as well as coping with chronic illness. Nearly all the patients (95%) reported that the contact was helpful.[3] Now the bad news! Many practitioners do not know that they are qualified and that they have the skills to be therapeutic; therefore they do not make the simple interventions that can be so highly effective. They often do not even ascertain that there is a problem. Studies have shown that although almost 60% of mental health care is provided in primary care settings, primary care providers fail to recognize up to two thirds of the emotional disorders manifested by their patients.[4,5] In one study, primary care providers failed to recognize six of seven patients with depressions, fifteen of eighteen with anxiety disorders, and all four drug or alcohol abusers.[6] In another, more recent study, only 19% of patients who visited primary care providers had their anxiety or depression identified and appropriately treated.[7] Instruments have been developed to alleviate these problems, but they are rarely used routinely with all patients.[8] It is critical to increase the probability of identifying a much greater proportion of these problems and making sure that they are adequately treated.

Although the literature is sparse and controversial, several studies have commented on the efficacy of psychotherapeutic techniques in primary care.[9-13] Counseling or psychotherapy by the primary care practitioner generally is considered to be appropriate by both patient and practitioner, but controlled, randomized trials are difficult to do. In one successful study, psychotherapy proved acceptable to both practitioner and patient, but the rigid protocol requiring exactly eight half-hour sessions, no psychiatric referrals, and no medications other than benzodiazepines cramped the practitioners' style. The eight-week limit proved ineffective in meeting the needs of patients with persistent psychological symptoms.[9]

Another structured program that was designed to teach practitioners specific behaviorally oriented treatment for depression was also unsuccessful.[10] Practitioners may not have favorable results with existing modalities of therapy, but there does seem to be agreement on the need to develop specific techniques and to train primary care practitioners to manage patients' psychological problems.[8-13] This objective is precisely what we would like to address.

Patients do talk to their primary care practitioners about their personal problems. Sometimes they are disappointed when the practitioner, after listening for a while, cuts them off without any acknowledgment or resolution. Our experience with family practice residents has shown that the residents frequently do not know what to say next or believe that enough time has been spent listening. So, after having spent some time letting the patient ventilate and nodding at seemingly appropriate places, they return abruptly to the business at hand: specifically the physical symptoms, the "safe" biomedical arena. In spite of this, we believe that many patients feel much better after talking to their doctor, even though the practitioner may not be aware of the therapeutic process in the interaction or of its impact on the patient.

Norman Cousins[14] has written much about the importance of the therapeutic interaction with the practitioner in promoting feelings of being cared for and in potentiating healing. In general, without the awareness of inherent skills and particular strategies, practitioners have a hard time dealing with the emotional aspects of patients' lives or illnesses. In one study, physicians expressed moderate self-confidence in their ability to prescribe medication for depression, panic disorder, and chronic anxiety, but they rated their psychotherapeutic abilities for these disorders much lower.[15] The simple techniques described in this text are designed to enhance both skills and confidence.

Writing in the *New England Journal of Medicine* in 1984, Benjamin[16] commented that with the then half-life of current medical knowledge at about five years and medical technology growing exponentially, many practitioners felt overwhelmed trying to keep up scientifically. Benjamin asserted that since the true healing skills are those of communication and caring, practitioners need to affirm the healing power of their words. He wrote the following:

The Greeks divided their healers into three categories: the "knife" doctor, the "herb" doctor, and the "word" doctor. Whereas the Greeks held them in balance, the low status today of the "word" doctors—the psychiatrists—indicates that we believe words are cheap if not useless. We are action oriented and get paid for performing procedures rather than for being—for doing rather than for talking. Western medicine, following the Cartesian dualism between mind and body, has become largely a somatic business. Words have been left behind in the rush to master chemistry. Emotions have been minimized in the reductionist effort to understand cells and genes.

All practitioners, whatever their specialty, can improve their therapy of the word. . . . The emotional condition of a patient is as basic as any single factor in the treatment of disease (p. 596).[16]

David Spiegel, M.D.,[17] writing an editorial entitled "Healing Words" in the *Journal of the American Medical Association* in 1999, also points out how traditional medicine has focused on the pathophysiology of disease and has ignored the psychophysiological reactions to disease processes. His final comment on the state of current research ends with ". . . it is not simply mind over matter, but it is clear that mind matters."[17] The important clinical question now becomes "How do we best use words to affect patients' minds?"

The separation of mind and body, as suggested in Chapter 1, has become an anachronistic paradigm. Because all physical illness has an emotional component and all emotional problems have some physical component, practitioners must respond in some way. Since publication of the first edition of *The Fifteen Minute Hour* many practitioners have reported that the techniques described in this text have helped them to respond empathetically, efficiently, and comfortably and that this has effectively promoted the patient's sense of well-being.[18-20] The healing dialogue between the practitioner and the patient constitutes the essence of a therapeutic intervention.

HOW TO BE A THERAPEUTIC PRACTITIONER

What are the characteristics of a therapeutic relationship? Let us look at a few of the more obvious factors.

Trust

The *sine qua non* of any therapeutic relationship is trust. Recent research confirms that ongoing doctor-patient relationships based on trust are critical for effective care.[21,22] Trust can be thought of as an assessment that a person is both competent to fulfill a promise and sincere in the desire to do so. If we (the practitioners) promise to do something that you (the patient) do not believe we are capable of doing, you will not trust us. Obviously, we cannot deliver on something that we are not able to do. On the other hand, if you do not believe that we are sincere in our desire to provide what we promise, again, you will not trust us. You do not have faith in our intentions. For trust to exist, you must be assured that we are both competent and genuine in our desire to be helpful.

Patients are able to specify the physician behaviors that are associated with trust.[23] Being caring and comforting and demonstrating competence and good communication are the behaviors most strongly associated with patient trust.[22,23]

When patients have confidence in the skill, integrity, and character of the practitioner, they feel free to expose personal aspects of their lives in order to receive help. Trust implies that patients feel assured that no harm will come from disclosing data about themselves, their lives, or those of their significant others. Patients expect that the information they share will be respected, understood, responded to, and kept confidential.[24]

There is also the expectation that practitioners will apply their training, experience, and skills to benefit their patients. In other words, patients believe in both the ability and the sincere desire of practitioners to care and provide help. Traditionally, trust has also implied a patient's expectation of not being rejected or abandoned. In primary care, the open-ended relationship, built over time, helps to build the patient's confidence. Unfortunately, the current health care delivery system often undermines continuity in relationships.[21,22]

In order for trust to develop, a history of successful encounters with this or other practitioners is essential. Successful, in this connotation, suggests that patients were able to get their needs met in previous encounters with practitioners. They have had positive experiences. It is, of course, possible that trust can exist without previous personal experience. Trust can be provided by association, such as when other persons who are trusted make a recommendation based on their experience. This is an example of social power, a topic to be discussed shortly.

These factors, singly and in concert, denote trust. The patient expects to be safe in the hands of the wise practitioner who is assumed to be capable of and committed to providing personal, ongoing, quality care and who will respect the patient's confidentiality.

Continuity

In primary care, an assumption is made that the practitioner's commitment to the patient has no defined end point.[25] The continuity of the relationship is thereby established. The personal practitioner does not treat the patient for just one illness episode but expects to follow the patient and attend to the patient's ongoing medical care. If the practitioner has known the patient and the patient's family over time, this simplifies the communication of particular aspects of any situation.

When the practitioner is familiar with the family structure, cultural background, and orientation toward health care and already knows many factors involved in a patient's personal situation, little time is required to be brought up to date. Also, the practitioner knows from the history of this particular patient's "care-seeking behavior" whether the patient tends to exaggerate or deny the severity of situations. Further, because of the continuity in the relationship, the practitioner can anticipate and follow critical transitions in the patient's life and can intervene in a timely and convenient fashion.

The salient point is that the relationship is preestablished. Even in a group practice, health maintenance organization (HMO), or prepaid plan, the patient "belongs" there. The records have been kept and provide continuity even if a different practitioner is seeing the patient. There is an expectation of consistent care and follow-up in the particular office, even if it is not with the same practitioner. The patient cannot be abandoned or rejected.

Support and Comfort

Competent adults are capable of taking care of themselves and of others who are dependent. However, when feeling down, besieged, or overwhelmed by physical or mental stressors, everyone experiences a need to be supported, nurtured, and comforted. Adults, children, practitioners, and patients are all vulnerable to the same forces. The more our resources feel depleted by virtue of the forces impinging on us, the more dependent we become. When this happens, support from others becomes an emergent need.

Practitioners, by profession, are seen as healers who provide care and nurture on demand. This expectation is brought by the patient and is generally met. By conducting a patient-centered interview, the practitioner focuses the interaction directly on the patient's needs.[26,27] Patients feel better after seeing the practitioner. As discussed in Chapter 1, the patient always gets something from the practitioner. The prescription or the written excuse may become the symbol of the sustenance that the patient seeks, but the caring may be entirely in the process. In any case, the patient asks for help and is open to receive whatever the practitioner is willing to provide. Since there is a positive expectation, there will be little resistance to experiencing the positive impact of quality caring. The patient assumes that the practitioner's training, intelligence, experience, and general wisdom will be devoted to the task of alleviating the patient's pain.

THE ISSUE OF POWER

Although practitioners are generally very aware of their power to affect life and death by the medical decisions they make, especially in the hospital setting, few practitioners have been exposed to the literature on social power. They tend to have little awareness of their impressive potential to influence certain aspects of their patients' attitudes and behavior.

What Is Social Power?

Social power has been defined as the potential that one person has to change the beliefs, attitudes, or behavior of another person.[28] Changing a patient's beliefs, attitudes, or behavior is the essence of the therapeutic intervention. In general, power can be defined as the potential or ability to satisfy needs. If we can satisfy our own needs, we have personal power. We are able to muster sufficient personal resources to get what we want and are not dependent on other people. If we are in a position to satisfy other people's needs or if they believe that we can satisfy their needs, they give us power. This type of power is generally referred to as social power. It enables one person to influence the behavior, thoughts, and feelings of another person.

There Is No Free Lunch

Social exchange theorists see all human relationships in terms of potential payoff.[29] Using this framework, all interpersonal relationships are seen as exchanges of behavior among people. Great stress is placed on the ability to provide rewards that cause behavior to be repeated. This common-sense approach suggests that people relate to other people only because they get something from the interaction. Those individuals who have commodities to trade have power.

Information and expertise are seen as highly valued commodities.[30] In this connection, Postman[31] points out that, to a large extent, the authority that adults have over children derives from their being the principal source of knowledge (information). Francis Bacon[32] was thus quite accurate when he asserted that "Knowledge is power."

Practitioners have a great deal of knowledge at their disposal, a *commodity* that they can use to relieve the distress of their patients. This knowledge is, however, only one source of the practitioner's power. Before we examine the many power resources at the disposal of the practitioner, it will be useful to distinguish between the concepts of attributed and manifest power.

Manifest Versus Attributed Power

When we say that we "give someone power," that generally implies that we hold them in high esteem and allow them to influence our behavior, our beliefs, and our attitudes. Social psychologists distinguish between *attributed* power and *manifest* power. Power is attributed to someone who is *believed* by others to have the potential to meet their needs. (Whether this is actually the case is totally irrelevant.) Manifest power, on the other hand, means that the ability to mobilize or withhold resources has been clearly demonstrated.

Practitioners have both types of power. First, they are given a great deal of attributed power. Patients respect practitioners (and sometimes fear them), believe them to have in-depth knowledge in many areas (some of which may actually be outside the practitioner's area of expertise), and expect to be influenced by them. Practitioners clearly have manifest power. This is demonstrated through ordering tests or hospitalizations, dispensing prescriptions, writing excuses, making referrals, filling out insurance or disability forms, providing reassurance, doing procedures, reporting seizures (which means taking away people's drivers' licenses), and reporting sexually transmitted or other contagious diseases, to mention only a few examples.

Types of Social Power

Although there are many ways to look at social power, the work of J.P.R. French, Jr., and B.H. Raven[28] clarifies the power base that operates in the practitioner-patient relationship. In the 1950s French and Raven analyzed a large body of empirical research on the outcome determinants of social power, that is, the psychological changes induced through the relationship between an influencer and an object. Their original formulation distinguished five specific types of power: reward, coercive, referent, legitimate, and expert. Later they sometimes added information as a separate source of social power.[30] They noted that having multiple types of power in a relationship increases the power base. Not surprisingly, they found that the more important the relationship, the stronger the base of the power that can be exerted by the influencer. Their recently expanded model of interpersonal effectiveness examined variables such as the motivation of the influencer, values, and norms, as well as the positive and negative effects that power bases may have.[30] We will discuss each of the original five sources of social power in relation to the practitioner-patient relationship. In our view, access to (medical) information is part of expert power and not a separate category and we assume that practitioners are motivated to use their power for the benefit of the patient.

Reward Power

The first type of social power distinguished by French and Raven, reward power, consists of the ability or resources to provide symbolic or material rewards: giving people what they want or need. In a practitioner-patient interaction, this might be attention, time, prescriptions, reassurance, approval, or advice. It can mean responding favorably to requests for information, medication, tests, procedures, or filling out administrative forms, that is, providing relief from disease, pain, or anxiety.

Coercive Power

Coercive power depends on the ability to respond to a person's behavior in a punitive way: to create negative or uncomfortable consequences. Coercive power is efficient in situations where one has a captive audience, but it is detrimental to the quality of relationships. Behavior that changes in response to coercion will revert to its natural form when supervision is removed. Coercive power is omnipresent in the practitioner's potential for giving disapproval, denying requests, prescribing aversive protocols, refusing to see patients or answer phone calls, and withholding permission for desired activities. The ineffectiveness of coercive power, in the absence of supervision, may well account for the dismal rate of patient compliance with medication regimens, especially when patients are dissatisfied with their relationships with their practitioners.[33-35]

Referent Power

The most potent of the interpersonal powers is probably referent power that is connected with a person's desire to identify with the other. The desire to identify is heightened by the attractiveness of the power source. The advertising industry spends billions of dollars capitalizing on the effectiveness of referent power. Currently, the image of golf star Tiger Woods has been brandished in dozens of advertisements promoting everything from cereal to sneakers or automobiles.[36] The positive feelings generated by the thought of associating oneself with a person or a group, connected by shared beliefs, are the most powerful and lasting way to influence a person.[37] Attitude or behavior change induced by referent power becomes internalized and self-maintaining quite rapidly. People want to like the role model, mentor, hero, or "admired other" in any way they can. They want to use the same products, engage in the same behaviors, and have the same opinions. It feels good. It makes them feel connected. That feeling further reinforces the power of the revered object.

Referent power can help ensure adherence in the outpatient setting. When the patient admires the practitioner and wants to both be like and be liked by the practitioner, cooperation is rewarding. Patients feel competent and virtuous when following directions. Patients also feel connected. Telling other people that "my doctor says I'm doing well," "understands that I feel awful," or "wants to see me again in a couple of weeks" makes patients feel good.

Legitimate Power

Legitimate power derives from perceptions that another person has an institutionalized right to exert influence. When a patient initiates a consultation, legitimate power is attributed to the practitioner. By contracting to pay for advice given, whether directly or through a third party, the patient acknowledges the legitimacy of the practitioner's right to give instructions. This right, in fact, becomes an obligation that the patient has instigated.

The more legitimate the power is perceived to be, the less resistance there is to the influence exerted. It is important to understand that the legitimacy derives from internalized values, where the patient accepts the practitioner as a valid authority with a right to prescribe standards. If the patient has ambivalent feelings toward authority growing out of a history of conflicts with coercive or overly demanding authority figures (e.g., father, teachers, bosses), there may well be a tendency to thwart the authority of the practitioner. Many patients have some problems with authority, so adherence to treatment recommendations is not always ensured, regardless of the legitimacy of the power. Subsequent chapters will discuss ways in which the practitioner can avoid power struggles smoothly.

Expert Power

The last type of power outlined by French and Raven[28] is expert power. Unquestionably, patients accept the practitioner as an expert in medical matters, including access to relevant information, and are therefore open to being influenced. The practitioner's word on psychological or social matters will also rarely be questioned, regardless of the actual level of the practitioner's knowledge. The patient attributes global expert power to the practitioner.

Clinical Application

Recent research on social power suggests that social power actually has a global factor.[38] Further, the more under stress and unsure about an issue a person feels, the more open that person is to help and suggestion. The more difficult the matter is to understand, the more persuasive the arguments of an expert are found to be. Conversely, when people hold firm beliefs or simplistic understandings, these must first be explored and acknowledged before counter arguments can be effective. Motivational interviewing capitalizes on these factors.[39] The practitioner helps the patient to sort out the positive and negative consequences of either changing or not changing a particular behavior. In this case, the practitioner demonstrates expertise through a process, rather than imposing a demand or issuing an edict for change.

It is interesting to note that information gets absorbed into a person's cognitive structure independent from its source. French and Raven[28] identify a "sleeper effect" that occurs when information is at first rejected by subjects because the source has a negative connotation (an expert perhaps, but not attractive or admired). Unfortunately, we have all experienced the power of negative advertising in political campaigns. Even supporters often accept distorted and unfavorable allegations about candidates because these allegations are heard repeatedly and the "facts" have become separated from their source. In experimental studies, subjects consistently forget the source of a communication faster than the content.[40] Hence, the power of rumors.

Primary care practitioners have tremendous potential for correcting erroneous or harmful psychosocial information previously internalized by patients. Negative information becomes part of a patient's belief system, affecting the patient's thoughts, attitudes, and behavior. Perhaps a significant authority figure has convinced the patient that he or she is unimportant as a person. This experience can produce poor self-esteem, a sense of helplessness, and a world view lacking in reinforcing encounters. The practitioner's expressed interest in the patient is incongruent with this view. Since the practitioner is perceived as a global source of social power, the therapeutic potential of intentionally made supportive statements and demonstrated respect cannot be minimized.

Conversely, practitioners have the power to undermine a patient's self-esteem and self-confidence. By talking down to the patient or discounting the patient's concerns, the practitioner reinforces the patient's low self-opinion. The manner in which evaluations or instructions are communicated becomes critical. For example, if a patient is concerned about a particular symptom, such as a vague pain, the practitioner's offhand instruction, "Don't worry about it!" not only discounts the patient and the patient's experience but also becomes an order that the patient cannot follow. This furthers lowers the patient's self-esteem and exacerbates anxiety. If, however, the practitioner says, "I have carefully examined you and I see no cause for concern" or "I'm not worried, this is quite normal," then the patient can infer that the condition is truly benign. The statement on the part of the practitioner regarding the practitioner's own lack of concern taps into feelings of identification. The patient thinks, "O.K., if the doctor is not worried, I don't have to worry either" or "My practitioner is an expert in these matters. Since she says it will go away by itself, it can't be serious. I guess I really don't have to worry."

People change their beliefs when they are convinced by information that, although different from their current understanding, presents a convincing picture based on the qualifications of the source providing the new information. But people change their beliefs only when they feel safe to do so and when they are ready.

Final Words on Power

The practitioner is at once a powerful, attractive, and credible source of information with great potential for effecting behavioral change in patients. The ability to manipulate others affords a measure of power and control that some practitioners find uncomfortable. J.W. Cone,[41] writing about mental health professionals, points out that although some clinicians may have some conflicts regarding issues of power and control, they appear to be unaware that they already hold a powerful upper hand in relation to their clients. Since this power already exists, Cone suggests that random, noncontingent, "unknowing" use has to be more frightening than the intentional application of the power in the service of the patient. This is precisely our point. The rich sources of power inherent in the clinician-patient relationship are a given. Our purpose is to raise the practitioner's level of awareness so that this power can be applied judiciously and skillfully toward the end of making patients feel better.

BUILDING ON EXISTING SKILLS

Every practitioner who knows how to talk with and listen to patients has the basic tools with which to provide psychological support. Essential skills in the medical interview consist of establishing rapport, eliciting information, clarifying the patient's problems, and then communicating the diagnosis and management plan. Talking with patients is primarily a theme-centered conversation, a conversation focused on the patient's concerns that includes relevant social, emotional, economic, and spiritual factors. This is the essence of the patient-centered interview.[26,27]

The Expanded Relationship

Practitioners are perhaps most skilled in the data collection aspect of the consultation. In our view, when gathering information dealing with the psychosocial aspect of the patient's problems, questions must be designed to help the patient become aware of the affective state being experienced. This includes the patient's assessment of current stressors and reactions to them, major concerns, and resources that can be mustered to reach some resolution. We are not conducting a psychiatric interview here. We do not advocate initiating a workup or an in-depth analysis of the patient's coping mechanisms. Although we expect that the practitioner would become aware of any major depressive or anxiety symptoms at this point, we are not interested in deriving a categorical differential diagnosis of mental disease. Instead, we assume that the patient is distressed and propose that the process of inquiry be structured to give the patient the opportunity to bring to awareness and reassess the situation in a more productive way. We are looking to normalize the patient's reaction. With this in mind, the data collection phase of the interview is specifically goal oriented, utilizing previously learned skills.

When practitioners gather data, they usually approach the patient in a logically organized way: What is troubling you? When did it start? What did you notice first? Please describe the symptoms. What makes it better? What makes it worse? What have you done that alleviates the discomfort? Information is gathered. It is prioritized and synthesized. When unexpected data are elicited, time is taken for reflection.[42] The practitioner attempts to get a comprehensive view, to avoid premature closure, and then to diagnose the problem. Having done this, the clinician explains the findings, communicates the management plan, and reassures the patient. These communication skills are all that is required to adequately treat the psychological aspects of the patient's problems. What is involved is simply a conscious, focused, deliberate application of the therapeutic agent: *the practitioner*. Therapeutic talk, or, as we prefer to label it, the therapeutic intervention, helps patients to identify problems, recognize when they started, discuss their effects, and figure out how they can be solved. It is the quality of the interaction between the clinician and the patient that promotes a positive effect on the patient's self-image and view of the world and empowers the patient to modify his or her story.

Communicating a Caring Attitude

The relationship between a *person* and the *other* is the most powerful therapeutic tool there is. How we relate to the other and the quality of the time we spend are often communicated most clearly nonverbally rather than verbally. Practitioners are aware of the value of eye contact, the powerful messages carried by body language, and the positive effect of active listening. It is the quality of the time given the patient that determines the therapeutic effect, not the absolute amount of time that the practitioner spends. Does the practitioner pay attention? Show interest? Concentrate? Every well-trained clinician should demonstrate these skills. These techniques have generally been *overlearned* and become automatic, having been performed repeatedly. When providing psychological support, as stated earlier, the practitioner must efficiently organize the data collection in order to clarify the problem for the patient. The patient needs to understand the situation in order to have power to affect it. It is not useful or time-effective for the practitioner to probe for details about how the situation evolved. It may satisfy the practitioner's curiosity but is often not therapeutic. It is not important to gather information about matters that the practitioner cannot control. It is, however, extremely useful for the patient to gain awareness about the response that is generated by the situation and to recognize the legitimacy of that response. Reassurance given by the practitioner consists of acknowledging to the patient that the symptoms, including the emergent emotional state, are appropriate. Patients then do not have to be upset about being upset or angry at themselves for feeling angry. They do not have to worry about being worried or be depressed about being depressed. The practitioner has diagnosed the situation as being a stressful one and pronounced the patient's reaction as logical and normal given the patient's perception. This is experienced as highly supportive. Later chapters will discuss ways to help patients modify their perceptions and reactions to stressors, but the first step is *always* to accept the patient's reaction.

Giving the patient positive attention of this type has an added therapeutic effect. Focusing on the psychosocial aspect of the patient's problems communicates genuine caring about the patient as a person. The healing is in the relationship. For most of us, attention from significant others is interpreted as a confirmation of our sense of worth and belonging. Children will do almost anything to get attention. We all know that if a child cannot get attention through some positive action, that child will act in some provocative fashion. Even a reprimand or a slap is better than no attention at all. It seems that there is a driving need to be attended to, even in negative ways. We need to feel connected to others, to be seen, heard, and acknowledged. By responding to the psychological needs of the patient in a positive and deliberate way, the practitioner therapeutically connects with the patient. By focusing the patient on potential solutions to problems or at least legitimizing the patient's current reaction, the practitioner enhances the patient's sense of autonomy and competence.

Perhaps there are those who will still question the practitioner's qualifications for providing therapeutic interventions or therapy of the word (i.e., psychotherapy). The simplest answer is that the opportunity is there. When patients feel bad enough to consult a practitioner, they may not even be aware of the specifics of what made them feel better; they only know that they feel better after the visit.

Eliciting the Context of the Visit

As discussed in Chapter 2, it is important to ascertain the reason that the patient has chosen this time to seek medical attention. It is, however, essential that this process not consume inordinate amounts of time. We have devised a simple and efficient protocol to explore the psychosocial context that has very specific, limited goals:

1. Raising the patient's awareness of the concomitant events that might be affecting his or her health status
2. Focusing the patient on the emotional state that is being experienced
3. Guiding the patient into specifying one aspect of the problem that is particularly troubling
4. Ascertaining the manner in which the patient is handling the experienced stress
5. Using active listening and providing an empathic response, which makes the patient feel validated

We ask four basic questions: What is going on? How do you feel about it? What troubles you the most? How are you handling that? Then we give the patient a response showing we have understood that there is a problem and that the patient is handling it as well as can be expected under the circumstances. It is crucial that the practitioner give this type of empathic response. As pointed out previously, no response or an abrupt change of topic may leave a patient feeling dissatisfied, even when the practitioner has spent time and given the patient the opportunity to ventilate about a problem. Anytime a patient expresses concerns about some issue, the practitioner *must* respond (if the practitioner wishes to be therapeutic). The phrase "That must be very difficult for you!" is extremely useful. We suggest that whenever a practitioner is at a loss for words after being presented with some complicated or painful problem, the automatic reply "That must be very difficult (or hard, painful, tiring, or discouraging) for you" is always appropriate. Coming from a powerful, attractive, knowledgeable source, such as the practitioner, it makes the patient feel affirmed.

Although the situation is tough, at least the response is reasonable. If this *is* a difficult situation, as understood by the clinician, the patient feels much better, not as subjectively out of control. Perhaps he or she is not as incompetent, worthless, or helpless as had been imagined, and perhaps it is not true that "nobody cares," since the clinician obviously cares. Hope is rekindled. The patient is no longer demoralized.

Tolerance for symptoms will be enhanced, and the healing capacity of the body will be facilitated.[43,44]

Often patients will go into great detail about their situations. By paraphrasing the patient's concerns and reactions to the problem, the practitioner demonstrates attentive listening and indicates that the patient has been understood. This interaction can make the patient feel both competent and connected. At the least, it will reduce the amount of detail and repetition in the patient's story. When the practitioner interjects that the situation obviously is difficult and he or she looks forward to hearing the outcome in follow-up, this allows the patient to move on. These easy-to-learn techniques constitute the essence of psychological support. Primary care practitioners are highly qualified to address these issues since they have both the skills and the opportunity to make effective therapeutic interventions.

A Brief Clinical Example

A 24-year-old woman visited the office, complaining of a sore throat and a mild earache that she had had for 10 days. The chart showed that there had been several previous visits for minor complaints and some evidence of mild postpartum depression. Her youngest child was currently 12 months old. There were two older children in the home. Questioning by the practitioner elicited no particular acute stress, just a general lack of enthusiasm. When asked about the progress of the baby, the patient brightened somewhat. The practitioner then suggested that taking care of an active one-year-old, especially at a busy time of the year and when she wasn't feeling well herself, must be very difficult. The patient gave a deep sigh, "Oh, how I wish that there was someone to take care of me." The practitioner responded, "I can understand that. It must be hard to constantly have to be in the role of nurturing Mom." He put his hand on her shoulder and gently guided her to the exam table. She smiled and relaxed. During the course of the exam he asked her to think about what *she* could do to carve out short periods of time to take care of herself.

This simple interaction did not solve the patient's problems or cure her "mild depression." However, as a result of the interaction, the patient obviously felt better, as shown by her affect. We assume that she interpreted the practitioner's comments as indicating that her response to her problems was reasonable and that therefore she was seen as a reasonable person. This lifted her spirits and her self-esteem. The practitioner also empowered her by giving her permission to plan for her own needs as well as those of her children.

SUMMARY

Since physical and emotional problems are substantially inseparable, adequate primary care medical treatment is really not possible without confronting the psychosocial dimension. Many patients already consider their practitioner their primary source of mental health care. The true healing skills are those of communication and caring. Primary care practitioners who establish relationships of trust, continuity, comfort, and support for their patients already have a base for making therapeutic interventions.

Social power is defined as the potential to influence the beliefs, attitudes, or behavior of another person. Practitioners have both manifest (demonstrated) power and attributed (assumed) power, which include reward, coercive, referent, legitimate, and expert power. Being powerful, attractive, and credible sources of information, practitioners have the potential to influence patients' behavior and effect permanent attitude change. Motivational interviewing engages a patient in exploring options for behavioral change. The power attributed to practitioners can be used with awareness, in the service of making patients feel better about themselves and their world.

Practitioners already have the necessary interviewing skills, such as data collection, organization, synthesis, and information communication, to establish quality relationships with patients that demonstrate attention, interest, and respect. Therapeutic interventions help patients to identify problems, recognize when they started, discuss their effects, and figure out how they can be solved. By establishing the context of the patient's visit and providing an empathic response, the practitioner can identify and help to mitigate the patient's distress.

REFERENCES

1. Locke, B.Z., & Gradner, E.P. Psychiatric disorders among the patients of general practitioners and internists. *Public Health Reports*, 1969, *84*, 167–173.
2. Üstun, T.B., & Von Korff, M. Primary mental health services: Access and provision of care. In Üstun, T.B., & Sartorius, N. (eds.) *Mental Illness in General Health Care: An International Study*. New York: Wiley, 1995.
3. Corney, R.H. A survey of professional help sought by patients for psychosocial problems. *British Journal of General Practice*, 1990, *40*, 365–368.
4. Kessler, D., Lloyd, K., Lewis, G., & Gray, D.P. Cross-sectional study of symptom attribution and recognition of depression and anxiety in primary care. *British Medical Journal*, 1999, *318*, 436–439.
5. Von Korff, M., Shapiro, S., Burke, J.D., Teitelbaum, M., Skinner, E.A., German, P.S., Turner, R.W., Klein, L., & Burns, B. Anxiety and depression in a primary care clinic: Comparison of diagnostic interview schedule, general health questionnaire, and practitioner assessments. *Archives of General Psychiatry*, 1987, *44*, 152–156.
6. Borus, J.F., Howes, M.J., Devins, N.P., Rosenberg, R., & Livingston, W.W. Primary health care providers' recognition and diagnosis of mental disorders in their patients. *General Hospital Psychiatry*, 1988, *10*, 317–321.
7. Young, A.S., Klap, R., Sherbourne, C., & Wells, K. The quality of care for depressive and anxiety disorders in the United States. *Archives of General Psychiatry*, 2001, *58*, 55–61.
8. Spitzer, R.L., Kroenke, K., Linzer, M., Hahn, S.R., Williams, J.B.W., deGruy, F.V., Brody, D., & Davies, M. Health-related quality of life in primary care patients with mental disorders: Results from the PRIME-MD 1000 Study. *Journal of the American Medical Association*, 1995, *274*, 1511–1517.
9. Brodaty, H., & Andrews, G. Brief psychotherapy in family practice: A controlled prospective intervention trial. *British Journal of Psychiatry*, 1983, *143*, 11–19.
10. Stepansky, P.E., & Stepansky, W. Training primary practitioners as psychotherapists. *Comprehensive Psychiatry*, 1974, *15*, 141–151.
11. Pierloot, R.A. The treatment of psychosomatic disorders by the general practitioner. *International Journal of Psychiatry in Medicine*, 1977–78, *8*, 43–51.
12. Pincus, H.A., Strain, J.J., Houpt, J.L., & Gise, L.H. Models of mental health training in primary care. *Journal of the American Medical Association*, 1983, *249*, 3065–3068.
13. Haug, T.T., Hellstrom, K., Blomhoff, S., Humble, M., Madshu, H.P., & Wold, J.E. The treatment of social phobia in general practice: Is exposure therapy feasible? *Family Practice*, 2000, *17*(2), 114–118.
14. Cousins, N. *The Healing Heart: Antidotes to Panic and Helplessness*. New York: W.W. Norton & Co., 1983.

15. Von Korff, M., & Myers, L. The primary care practitioner and psychiatric services. *General Hospital Psychiatry*, 1987, *9*, 235–240.

16. Benjamin, W.W. Sounding board: Healing by the fundamentals. *New England Journal of Medicine*, 1984, *311*, 595–597.

17. Spiegel, D. Healing words: Emotional expression and disease outcome. *Journal of the American Medical Association*, 1999, *281*(14), 1328–1329.

18. Nutter, D.W. Letter re "Windows of opportunity to address patients' concerns: Too small too few?" *Journal of the American Medical Association*, 1993, *270*, 1195.

19. McCullock, M., Ramesar, S., & Peterson, H. Psychotherapy in primary care: The BATHE technique. *American Family Physician*, 1998, *57*, 2131–2134.

20. Conley, S.C. Resident and student voice: Deep waters. *American Family Physician*, 2001, *63*, 383–384.

21. Murphy, J., Chang, H., Montgomery, J.E., Rogers, W.H., & Safran, D.G. The quality of physician-patient relationships: Patients' experiences 1996–1999. *Journal of Family Practice*, 2001, *50*(2), 123–129.

22. Safran, D.G., Montgomery, J.A., Chang, H., Murphy, J., & Rogers, W.H. Switching doctors: Predictors of voluntary disenrollment from a primary physician's practice. *Journal of Family Practice*, 2001, *50*(2), 130–136.

23. Thom, D.H., & Stanford Trust Study Physicians. Physician behaviors that predict trust. *Journal of Family Practice*, 2001, *50*(4), 323–328.

24. Mechanic, D., & Meyer, S. Concepts of trust among patients with serious illness. *Social Science and Medicine*, 2000, *51*(5), 657–668.

25. McWhinney, I.R. *A Textbook of Family Medicine*. New York: Oxford University Press, 1989.

26. Levenstein, J.H., McCracken, E.C., McWhinney, I.R., Stewart, M.A., & Brown, J.B. The patient-centered clinical method. I. A model for clinician-patient interaction in family practice. *Family Practice*, 1986, 3, *24–30*.

27. Brown, J.B., Stewart, M.A., McCracken, M.C., McWhinney, I.R., & Levenstein, J.H. The patient centered clinical method: Definition and application. *Family Practice*, 1986, *3*, 75–79.

28. French, J.P.R., Jr., & Raven, B.H. The bases of social power. In Cartwright, D., & Zander, A. (eds.) *Group Dynamics: Research and Theory*, 3rd ed. New York: Harper & Row, 1968.

29. Kelley, H.H., & Thibaut, J.W. *Interpersonal Relationships*. New York: John Wiley & Sons, 1978.

30. Raven, B. A power/interaction model of interpersonal influence: French and Raven thirty years later. *Journal of Social Behavior & Personality*, 1992, *7*(2), 217–244.

31. Postman, N. *The Disappearance of Childhood*. New York: Delacorte Press, 1982.

32. Bacon, F. Meditationes sacrae. Cited in Bartlett, J. *Familiar Quotations*, 13th ed. Boston: Little, Brown & Co., p. 118.

33. Becker, M.H. Patient adherence to prescribed therapies. *Medical Care*, 1985, *23*, 539–555.

34. Meichenbaum, D., & Turk, D. *Facilitating Treatment Adherence: A Practitioner's Guidebook*. New York: Plenum, 1987.

35. Brody, D.S. An analysis of patient recall of their therapeutic regimens. *Journal of Chronic Diseases*, 1980, *33*, 57–63.

36. Kukcevich, D. Forbes faces: Tiger Woods, *Forbes*, November 14, 2000. Downloaded 6/12/01.

37. Kelman, H.C. Compliance, identification and internalization: Three processes of attitude change. *Journal of Conflict Resolution*, 1958, *2*, 51–60.

38. Nesler, M.S., Aguinis, H., Quigley, B.M., Lee, S., & Tedeschi, J.T. The development and validation of a scale measuring global social power based on French and Raven's power taxonomy. *Journal of Applied Social Psychology*, 1999, *29*(4), 750–771.

39. Rollnick, S., & Miller, W.R. What is motivational interviewing? *Behavioural and Cognitive Psychotherapy*, 1995, *23*, 325–339.

40. Underwood, J., & Pezdek, K. Memory suggestibility as an example of the sleeper effect. *Psychonomic Bulletin & Review*, 1998, *5*, 449–453.

41. Cone, J.W. Formal models of ego development: A practitioner's response. In Datan, N., & Ginsberg, L.H. (eds.) *Life-Span Developmental Psychology: Normative Life Crises*. New York: Academic Press, 1975.

42. Schon, D.A. *Educating the Reflective Practitioner*. San Francisco: Jossey-Bass, 1987.

43. Cassel, J. The contribution of the social environment to host resistance. *American Journal of Epidemiology*, 1976, *104*, 107–123.

44. House, J.S., Landis, K.R., & Umberson, D. Social relationships and health. *Science*, 1988, *241*, 540–545.

CHAPTER 4

Principles and Strategies for Therapeutic Interventions

This chapter will clarify exactly what we mean by the term "practical therapeutic interventions." It is using the practitioner-patient relationship and the process of the therapeutic encounter to precipitate change in patients' views of themselves and their options. In our view what we are talking about is "psychotherapy." In our many workshops based on *The Fifteen Minute Hour* practitioners often tell us that they feel uncomfortable with the word "psychotherapy." They prefer to use the word "counseling." The distinction we make is that counseling refers to giving patients suggestions or advice, whereas psychotherapy, or therapeutic intervention, implies that we are deliberately using psychological techniques to attempt to modify how patients view themselves, their world, and their options in that world. Practitioners should be aware that words have the same potential as procedures to markedly affect patients' views of their current reality.

J.D. Frank,[1] in the revised edition of *Persuasion and Healing*, defines psychotherapy as influence characterized by three elements: first, a trained, socially sanctioned healer, whose healing powers are accepted by the sufferer; second, a sufferer who seeks relief from the healer; and finally a circumscribed series of contacts between the healer and the sufferer. He suggests that "the efficacy of psychotherapeutic methods lies in the shared belief of the participants that these methods will work." It is our contention that contacts between patients and primary care practitioners whose intention is to provide psychological support fulfill these criteria.

As pointed out in earlier chapters, psychological factors both predispose the patient to illness and affect recovery from illness. Therefore interventions or techniques designed to decrease psychological pain or dysfunction have a critical role in good medical treatment. Psychotherapy is the treatment of emotional, behavioral, personality, or psychiatric disorders, primarily by communication with the patient as an alternative or in addition to treatments utilizing chemical or physical measures. Psychotherapy can be understood as a process that uses a variety of verbal and nonverbal messages to empower patients. It enables patients to increase their trust in themselves and others, validates their feelings, enhances their sense of self-esteem, diminishes their feelings of isolation or depression, and helps them develop a sense of purpose and put it into action. We will identify specific, practical techniques that can be effectively incorporated into the brief primary care office visit.

Psychotherapy consists of the things we say—and the process of how we say them—that make the patient feel better. Our interaction with the patient, the therapeutic talk, has an ameliorating effect on the patient's distress. Different schools of psychiatry and psychology will claim that training and supervision in their particular method of psychotherapy are the critical factors in precipitating the change in self-image, world view, emotional response, or overt behavior that is associated with a successful outcome in psychotherapy. We maintain that certain universal influences can be used therapeutically and that understanding these dynamics and applying them intentionally potentiate healing.

HUMAN BEINGS TELL STORIES

Every one of us makes assumptions about the nature of the world based on our personal experiences starting in early childhood. Much of this process is out of the level of awareness. Then, as one talented psychotherapist puts it:

> We perpetuate these conditioned ways of perceiving the world through repetitive stories we tell ourselves about "the way things are." These kinds of stories are mental fabrications, judgments or interpretations that put what is happening into a familiar framework. Usually we do not recognize these stories as our own invention; instead, we believe that they represent reality.[2]

The more neurotic people are, the more distorted their world view and the more limited their stories. Patients never question these stories about who they are and what they are capable of, yet the stories act to place limits on subsequent experiences. Patients are not aware that this is not the only way to look at the world, themselves, or their situation.

PSYCHOTHERAPY MEANS EDITING THE STORY

Psychotherapy can affect the stories that patients tell themselves. Perhaps the simplest definition for psychotherapy is what we do to "fix" patients' maps of the world so that they can figure out the way to go to get what they want. Research has overwhelmingly demonstrated the effectiveness of psychotherapy over placebo or no-treatment approaches, but little evidence demonstrates the superiority of one type of therapy over another.[3,4] Certain approaches, however, lend themselves more effectively to specific types of clinical situations, as discussed later.

Our major concern is to define and modify those therapeutic features that work, regardless of the "brand name." The most effective techniques are generic. Our mission is to try to clarify what works, how to do it, and what we want to accomplish. Just exactly what are our goals?

THERAPEUTIC GOALS

Most simply put, the goal of therapeutic interventions is to make patients feel better, specifically to lower levels of distress and combat feelings of being overwhelmed. As pointed out in Chapter 2, when patients feel overwhelmed by the circumstances of their lives or their reaction to those circumstances, they develop a wide range of somatic and psychological symptoms. The most common symptoms from which patients suffer are anxiety and depression, which often occur simultaneously and may be accompanied by other somatic manifestations.[5-7] These symptoms develop because of patients' interpretations of their situation (their stories about the situation), not because of the situation proper. However, regardless of etiology, the experience of the symptoms further compromises patients' coping ability.

Patients Go on *Tilt*

When patients' coping ability becomes overextended they cease functioning effectively, a condition we label as *tilt*. The goal of psychotherapeutic intervention is to make the patient feel better so that the patient can function better, or go off *tilt*. Feeling better in this connotation relates to the emotional or mental state of the patient.

Specifically, we are concerned with patients' *perceived* personal power to deal with the circumstances of their lives. The sense of control has been shown to be the key factor in maintaining physical and mental health.[8] When people perceive themselves to be in control, whether they are or not, they function better. Perceived control has been shown to have a direct effect on autonomic reactivity and immune response.[8] Perceived control enables a person to function better in response to demands from both the internal and external environments. At the least, it improves coping, which also helps to restore the person's equilibrium, resulting in greater feelings of competence and belonging. Basically, our therapeutic goal is to help patients regain their sense of competence, so that they feel empowered to affect the course of their lives.

Why It Is Important to Have the Patient Back in Control

Once the patient's psychological state improves, the patient not only will be able to function better in the realms of interpersonal relations and job performance, but also will be more effective in mobilizing the body's defenses in response to existent or potential disease.[9,10] The patient with an enhanced sense of well-being will sleep better, have a healthier appetite, and maintain a more reasonable flow of energy. In contrast to the vicious cycle of demoralization, depression, and compromised immune response leading to disease and further demoralization, the body's healthy defenses will be engaged, leading to an enhanced sense of personal competence and improved ability to resist disease.[11]

Often the psychotherapeutic intervention will cause patients to make positive changes in their assumptive world view, meaning that it will allow them to edit their stories and add new chapters. This altered belief system then precipitates new ways of thinking and behaving that result in more satisfactory experiences, providing a natural reinforcement mechanism and instigating a benevolent circle.[12] A third-year family practice resident described the following case:

The patient is a 62-year-old white male whom I had been seeing routinely for blood pressure checks. He has a history of hypertension and peptic ulcer disease. He is a rather stoic person who generally keeps his feelings to himself, and, as I found out, "somatizes" and develops symptoms. After seeing him several times for vague and persistent abdominal discomfort, I persisted in knowing what was going on in his life. He mentioned problems at work and at home and then unexpectedly added that the combination had made him impotent. When I asked him how that made him feel, he at first denied that it had any effect but then complained of headaches. Questioned about what troubled him the most, the patient said it was his impotence because he could not satisfy his wife, even with her reassurance that "it doesn't bother her." I then asked how he was handling the stress. He replied that he gets up and "walks it off." After assuring the patient that this must be very difficult, I taught him some progressive relaxation techniques to help manage his stress and after tapering all medications that could contribute to his impotence referred him to a urologist. The interesting thing is that in all subsequent visits he expects to be questioned about his stressors and considers it part of his treatment. Unfortunately, at present he is still impotent. Although there are no medical contraindications, he has repeatedly declined a prescription for sildenafil (Viagra), but there are no more complaints of abdominal pain or headaches.

Supportive Therapy

Traditionally, a broad distinction has been made between supportive psychotherapy and explorative psychotherapy. Supportive therapy is designed to restore premorbid or optimal functioning (making the patient feel *competent and connected*), whereas explorative therapy is concerned with uncovering personality patterns to understand the etiology of disorders (why the patient does not feel *competent and connected*). Techniques promoted by proponents of supportive therapy include abreaction (catharsis: giving patients a chance to talk about the problem), dependency (being there for the patient), exploration of symptomatology, encouragement of new more productive behavior, and efforts at resolution through clarification. Basically, to be effective, all therapeutic interventions must be supportive, *with the goal of helping patients to feel competent and connected.*

Explorative Therapy

In explorative therapy the patient's behavior and feelings are examined from a historical perspective. Jerome Frank[12] has pointed out that if we mean by cure that we can eradicate the cause of illness, the "features of the patient's illness that psychotherapy can cure directly would be those caused by stress-producing distortions in the patient's assumptive world. Since the patient is an open psychobiological system, correction of these distortions would inevitably be reflected in changes in the neurophysiology of the central nervous system" (p. 17).[12]

We cannot stress too strongly that insight or understanding by itself has no practical benefit. P. Watzlawick, J.H. Weakland, and R. Fisch,[13] in their book *Change: Principles of Problem Formation and Problem Resolution*, make the following point:

Everyday experience, not just clinical practice, shows that there can be change without insight. In fact, very few behavioral or social changes are accompanied, let alone preceded, by insight into the vicissitudes of their genesis. It may, for instance, be that the insomniac's difficulty has its roots in the past: his tired, nervous mother may habitually have yelled at him to sleep and to stop bothering her. But while this kind of discovery may provide a plausible and at times even very sophisticated explanation of a problem, it usually contributes nothing towards its solution (p. 86).[13]

In a brilliant footnote these authors argue as follows:

Such empirical findings . . . (must be) thought through to their logical conclusions. There are two possibilities: (1) The causal significance of the past is only a fascinating but inaccurate myth. In this case, the only question is the pragmatic one: How can desirable change of present behavior be most efficiently produced? (2) There is a causal relationship between the past and present behavior. But since past events are obviously unchangeable, either we are forced to abandon all hope that change is possible, or we must assume that—at least in some significant respects—the past has influence over the present only by way of a person's present interpretation of past experience. If so, then the significance of the past becomes a matter not of "truth" and "reality," but of looking at it here and now in one way rather than another. Consequently, there is no compelling reason to assign to the past primacy or causality in relation to the present, and this means that the reinterpretation of the past is simply one of many ways of possibly influencing present behavior. In this case, then, we are back at the only meaningful question, i.e., the pragmatic one: How can desirable change of present behavior be produced most efficiently? (p. 86).[13]

So, contrary to conventional wisdom, *why* people are behaving in a particular manner is irrelevant. If the behavior is destructive, it is important to help them to change it. (In some cases, very intellectual types may feel that they must understand why before they can bring themselves to change—but in the final analysis it is their decision to make a change that is effective, not understanding why they behaved the way they did in the first place.)

FIVE COMMON ELEMENTS IN EFFECTIVE PSYCHOTHERAPY

The field of the psychotherapies includes a wide variety of modalities and orientations. There is long-term, short-term, individual, group, couple, and family therapy. In any of these modalities, the orientation can be behavioral, interpersonal, psychoanalytical, client-centered, gestalt, transactional, dynamic, cognitive, existential, reality-oriented, schema-focused, rational emotive, neurolinguistic, or eclectic, to mention only a few. Regardless of theoretical orientation, certain basic principles and strategies are associated with the therapeutic change process.[14]

As practitioners, when we make therapeutic interventions, we intentionally apply these generic forces.

The Expectation of Receiving Help

Common to all psychotherapeutic modalities is the initially induced expectation that the therapy will be helpful. Jerome Frank[15,16] has repeatedly pointed out that patients seek therapy because they are feeling helpless, hopeless, and demoralized. He has specifically defined the demoralization commonly experienced by patients as "a state of subjective incapacity plus distress. The patient suffers from a sense of failure, loss of self-esteem, feelings of hopelessness or helplessness and feelings of alienation or isolation. These are often accompanied by a sense of mental confusion, which the patient may express as a fear of insanity" (p. 19).[12] The expectation that help is imminent helps to lift the patient from the depths of demoralization.

The Therapeutic Relationship

The second general principle associated with all psychotherapeutic modalities is the client's or patient's participation in a therapeutic relationship. This relationship exists for the sole purpose of fostering the well-being of the patient. A contract (or understanding) is made in which another person agrees to engage with the patient in a manner that fosters the expression of feelings and concerns in an accepting atmosphere. This contract for caring and concern is the core of therapy. It is the nature of the relationship that determines the efficacy of the healing process. This is true whether we are discussing the classical analyst who listens and occasionally interprets, the Rogerian therapist who gives nonjudgmental reflections to the client, or the reality therapist who expects the patient to honor commitments and make no excuses. Regardless of theoretical orientation, it is the connection—the special relationship with the practitioner who communicates understanding and respect for the patient, takes the patient seriously, and is devoted to the patient's welfare—that is the generic healing component.

Obtaining an External Perspective

The third factor found in all psychotherapies is giving patients the opportunity to obtain an external or new perspective on their problems. By bringing their perceptions of their situation to a person not directly involved, patients are exposed to alternative interpretations, are made aware of potential options, and learn something about how other people might react to a similar situation. The external perspective affords patients an opportunity to check their possibly inaccurate perceptions of reality, the stories they are telling themselves about what is going on in their life. If the listener does not get upset when hearing about the outrageous situation that the patient describes, there may yet be a reasonable way to react. Perhaps there is some hope after all.

Encouraging Corrective Experiences

All psychotherapeutic modalities encourage corrective experiences. The definition of the corrective experience may vary according to the theoretical orientation of the practitioner, but until insights are put into practice and actually change how patients relate to themselves, their world, and the significant others in their lives, no healing occurs. The practitioner acts as consultant and cheerleader, encouraging patients to think and behave in new ways that result in a sense of enhanced well-being. This is the essence of a corrective experience. Patients are coached to react to situations in less destructive ways. The benefits of this improved behavior include gaining greater satisfaction from their interactions with others, which then promotes further gains.

Providing the Opportunity to Test Reality Repeatedly

The last principle common to all psychotherapies is the opportunity to test reality repeatedly. Patients' judgments of others, including others' intentions, are often quite inaccurate. These judgments are part of the story that the patients constantly repeat to themselves. An objective listener can confirm the reasonableness of the patients' reactions, challenge the accuracy of patients' conclusions, and/or suggest alternate interpretations. By examining their possibly faulty assumptions, patients are able to get a more accurate view of personal patterns of behavior, strengths, and vulnerabilities. Emotional and behavioral limitations will be reexamined. Certain goals that may previously have been judged as unattainable (not on the map) may now be seen as possible. Conversely, through repeated reality testing, unrealistic expectations are modified to become more reasonable and hence more likely to be satisfied. Often, patients need repeated confirmation that the experience of making changes can be difficult, painful, and slow.

STARTING WHERE THE PATIENT IS

Before we describe specific psychotherapeutic techniques, we would like to discuss three theoretical areas that provide important guidelines for understanding and modifying patients' reactions to their circumstances. Our focus will be on the importance of language in the creation of reality, explanatory styles used to explain causality, and the sense of self-efficacy.

Language and the Story

In *The Structure of Magic*[17] R. Bandler and J. Grinder, the founders of neurolinguistic programming (NLP), describe the process people use to record their experiences and create their maps (or stories). The basic premise is that there is an irreducible difference between the actual world and our experience of it. Each of us creates a mental representation of the world based on our experience. This representation (model or map) subsequently governs our behavior. Since no two people have identical experiences, we all have different models of the world. Bandler and Grinder's contribution was to clarify the process by which these models are built.

From birth we are bombarded with huge amounts of stimuli. In order to process information effectively, we tend to organize it in specific ways, lumping together similar experiences and creating rules and categories. All information about the world gets processed through our various senses: visual, auditory, and kinesthetic. In attending to the world, each of us chooses a predominant sense and communicates this in the descriptive language we use. The visually oriented person will "see what you mean," the auditory dominant person will "hear you," and the kinesthetic person will "feel" that he or she understands. Successful therapists automatically respond in the same mode as the patient.

We now return to the map. Why is it that some people are able to respond creatively and cope productively with most of life's problems, whereas other people generally perceive few options in any situation? The second group seems to be using an impoverished map. In the face of the multifaceted, rich, and complex world we inhabit, Bandler and Grinder wondered how people maintained such limited models, even when these models caused them so much pain. The linguists went on to describe three perceptual mechanisms that block growth and prevent the integration of new experience: generalization, deletion, and distortion.

Generalization is necessary for organizing information and coping with the world. The overwhelming amount of information received every second by our senses must be sorted into manageable categories. Generalizing from the experience of being burned to refrain from touching a hot stove has survival value, but generalizing that stoves are dangerous and must be avoided is dysfunctional. Having been discouraged from expressing negative feelings as a child, a person may generalize that it is bad to express any feelings. This may further generalize to the person thinking that simply having feelings is bad.

Based on early generalizations, people *delete* (i.e., selectively filter out) experiences that counter their established views. For example, people block themselves from hearing messages of caring that conflict with their generalizations of being unlovable. People who think of themselves as stupid will not be able to hear comments that attest to their intelligence. They will question the other's motive and accuracy of perception. Hence, we recommend the clinician say, "My, that was a difficult problem," instead of "Gee, you did that well."

The third modeling process involves *distortion* of sensory data to conform to preexisting notions. People hear and see what they expect to hear and see. Given a variety of experiences, people notice only those aspects that confirm their established sense of themselves and the universe. This results in their personal creation of their map, their story, or, as currently labeled, their "schema."

The process of therapy challenges the generalizations, deletions, and distortions inherent in the patient's experience of reality and thereby introduces changes into the patient's model of the world. Using cognitive therapy the clinician directly confronts these issues.

Making a Therapeutic Intervention

For the primary care practitioner what is important to remember is that language is used to organize the story about what is happening in the world and how the patient feels about it. Language affects how the patient represents past experiences in the present, including rules about what behaviors are acceptable and what behaviors are not acceptable. Language also structures what patients tell themselves about the future and what is likely to happen. Language is also the medium for making corrections in the story. That's what makes the practitioner's words so powerful.

In challenging generalizations, absolutes, such as *always, never, everyone,* and *no one,* need to be questioned; for example, "You're absolutely always in pain?" "No one has ever accepted your ideas?" "You've never done anything right?"

Deletions are exhibited through leaving gaps in expressions. In challenging deletions, it is useful to get patients to specify missing information. When a patient says, "I'm afraid," the practitioner must respond, "Of what *specifically* are you afraid?" The response to "I'm not good enough" is "In *what way* are you not good enough?" or "Specifically, *for what* are you not good enough?" Another possible challenge would be "How good is good enough?"

Distortions often occur when patients change verbs into nouns, such as "relating" to "relationship" or "deciding" to "decision." Bandler and Grinder point out that when we turn a "process" into an "event," which is then seen as unchangeable, this is limiting, guilt-producing, and destructive:

> Patient: "I really regret my decision."
> The response: "What stops you from changing your mind now?"
> Patient: "My relationship is a disaster."
> The response: "Is there a way you can respond to your partner in a different way?"

In challenging models, the practitioner questions not only absolutes but also imposed limits (the can'ts, shoulds, musts, and impossibilities—"Why not?") and imposed values (the rights, wrongs, "goods," and "bads") and in the process helps the patient to create a richer representation of possibilities.

Explanatory Style

We have been talking about the importance of patients' stories, their accounts of their experiences, in influencing their subsequent perceptions. There is a growing body of research that empirically establishes the connection between people's explanations of why something happened and their subsequent emotional and physical state. Martin Seligman and his colleagues, building on his work on *learned helplessness*,[18] conducted an innovative series of studies that found having a "pessimistic explanatory style" not only was associated with depressive symptoms but also was a risk factor in predisposing individuals to subsequent depressions when faced with negative situations.[19] This research focused on the explanations given for the occurrence of bad events in people's lives. Using data from interviews, questionnaires, and a technique of content analysis of verbal explanations (CAVE) that accommodates to use historical data such as diaries, letters, transcripts, and other records, these researchers were able to tie explanatory style to health outcomes and longevity.[20]

Explanatory style encompasses three dimensions: (1) whether the event is internally or externally caused—personal responsibility or attributed to others or circumstances;

Table 4–1   Examples of Stories Explaining Why My Checking Account Is Overdrawn

	EXPLANATORY STYLE			
	INTERNAL		EXTERNAL	
	STABLE	UNSTABLE	STABLE	UNSTABLE
GLOBAL	I'm incapable of doing anything right.	I've had the flu for several weeks. I let everything go.	All institutions chronically make mistakes.	Around the holidays everything gets fouled up.
SPECIFIC	I always have trouble figuring my balance.	The one time I didn't enter a check, my account gets overdrawn.	This bank has always used antiquated techniques.	I'm surprised! My bank has never made a mistake before.

From Peterson, C., & Seligman, M.E.P. Causal explanations as a risk factor for depression: Theory and evidence, *Psychological Review*, 1984, *91*, 349.

(2) whether the cause is stable or unstable—this is something that will always be this way, or this is something that happened on this occasion; and (3) whether the event is global or specific—this is something that happens with everything or just with this type of situation. Table 4–1 illustrates the range of stories to explain why a checking account might have been overdrawn using these dimensions.

Consistently using explanations from the internal, stable, global box puts people at risk for both morbidity and mortality. Optimists live longer than pessimists.[21,22] They stay healthier.[23] Grant study subjects (see Chapter 2) who exhibited the pessimistic explanatory style during their college days had significantly more cardiac pathological findings 35 years later than did their more optimistic colleagues.[24] Pessimistic explanatory style has even been directly linked to cell-mediated immunity in an elderly population.[25] When all three negative factors are present, the individual feels helpless, hopeless, and overwhelmed, leading to physical and emotional consequences.

Responding to Explanatory Style

Explanatory style is a fairly stable trait.[26] Although only habitual use of the pessimistic explanatory style has been shown to lead to negative health consequences, questioning this destructive manner of thinking can be highly therapeutic. It is useful to listen carefully to patients' explanations for the bad things that happen to them and to challenge internal, stable, and global causation. Is it really their fault, or did external factors or other people influence the event (internal)? Does this really happen all the time and is it likely to continue, or might this change in the future; and what can be done to facilitate that change (stable)? Does this really happen in all areas of the patient's life, or is this an area of particular weakness (global)? These questions may help patients recognize their exaggerated pessimistic assumptions and create conditions that may lead to positive change.

THE POWER INHERENT IN THE WORD OR CONCEPT OF "YET"

Helping patients edit their stories does not have to be time-consuming or complicated. The word "yet" is a very important therapeutic tool. When a patient makes a statement about his or her inability to do something, the practitioner can counter, "You have not been able to do that *yet!*" or "Up to now, this has been difficult for you." These statements imply that this is not a stable situation. This simple intervention is actually psychotherapy. It has the potential to change the patient's view. The same technique can be used to respond to statements when patients complain that they "always" have a certain difficulty. The response: "Yes, that has been your experience so far. You have not solved it yet."

We encourage practitioners to consistently question notions that problems have a stable quality, since they may be resolved at some future time, and to suggest that certain critical factors involved in a situation are not under the patient's control and that there are aspects of the patient's life that are successful, in spite of the fact that there may be problems with some particular aspects. When practitioners consistently point out that problems do not necessarily have internal, stable, and global causes, patients may be encouraged to develop a more positive explanatory style.

The Sense of Self-Efficacy

In treating dysfunctional behavior we have found that cognitive processes, termed "stories," determine and maintain habitual functioning. Successful change depends on changing habits and is performance-oriented, meaning that it relates to doing something. Albert Bandura[27] first postulated the concept of *self-efficacy* as a way of explaining the reciprocal relationship between performance and the cognitive assessment of the likelihood of success. People's beliefs in their ability to succeed at something determine whether behavior is initiated, the amount of effort that is expended, and how long that effort is sustained when obstacles or adverse reactions are experienced. These beliefs are based on past performance, vicarious experience, physiological and psychological states, and feedback regarding the current performance. The concept of self-efficacy is very useful for understanding and predicting behavior and also for providing a strategy to induce change. A diverse and rapidly expanding medical literature documents the importance of self-efficacy. This includes the relationship between self-efficacy and chronic obstructive pulmonary disease (COPD),[28] return to work after angioplasty,[29] mediating disability related to chronic pain,[30] recovery from orthopedic surgery,[31] quality of life of cancer patients,[32] and maintaining physical and role functions in coronary heart disease (CHD),[33] to mention only a few. The bottom line is that patients' predictions of what they will do are the most reliable indicators of what will transpire. If patients think that they are able to do something, they will try. If they fail at first, they will continue to try because based on past experiences, they believe it is only a question of time until they will succeed. Conversely, if patients have a low sense of self-efficacy and do not expect to be able to succeed, they may or may not try, their effort will be limited, and on encountering difficulties, their tendency will be to give up since their expectation is of failure anyway.

There is little sense in prescribing a nicotine patch to help patients stop smoking until those patients believe they can kick the habit, redefine themselves as nonsmokers, and develop healthy activities to substitute for the smoking urge. The sense of self-efficacy is not just a cognitive estimate of potential performance based on perceptions of past accomplishment but is directly instrumental in enhancing performance.[34]

Bandura's work is valuable because it points to mechanisms that can positively affect the sense of self-efficacy. These include structuring successes so the efficacy expectation is modified, providing vicarious experiences, creating supportive environments, and using verbal persuasion to change patients' views of the task or themselves.

The Power of Positive Illusions

Traditional concepts of mental health have proposed that well-adjusted individuals have a relatively accurate perception of themselves and their ability to control important aspects of their lives. There is now an impressive body of literature that suggests that having positive illusions about the self, personal control, and the future not only enhances performance but also results in a wide range of positive mental health outcomes.[35] This, too, can be seen as evidence that people's stories are the basis of self-fulfilling prophecies.

In summary, positive information that the practitioner provides about the patient or about a task (that the patient has just not been successful yet) may affect the patient's sense of self-efficacy and encourage the patient to engage in beneficial behavior change. The resulting positive outcome then further enhances the patient's sense of self-efficacy. Subsequently, the patient's story about what can be accomplished changes. The therapeutic intervention has been successful.

USEFUL TECHNIQUES FROM A VARIETY OF SOURCES

Having outlined the major generic therapeutic components common to all psychotherapeutic interventions and sketched some interesting models that explain mechanisms involved in patient's dysphoric experiences, we will now focus on therapeutic pearls from a variety of orientations. There are clearly some techniques that are more effective than others, some that are easier to learn than others, and some that lend themselves more comfortably to a therapeutic encounter within a 15-minute framework.

Psychodynamics in Brief

In general, people are simpler than insight schools imply but more complex than behavioral models suggest. By simpler we mean that a limited number of supportive techniques are highly effective, and by complex we mean that people's reactions are determined by a multitude of factors both in and out of awareness.

The unique contribution of psychodynamic theories is pointing out the hidden agendas that pervade interpersonal relationships, and the effect of maladaptive personal responses, influenced by past experiences, that are projected onto current relationships. The way patients define themselves as loving or hateful, competent or inadequate, is an ongoing process, a story that they are telling themselves based on judgments they have made over time. Some of this process is purely symbolic and unconscious, and some is within the awareness of the patient. Since much of this behavior is demonstrated in relation to the practitioner, an opportunity is created to bring these dynamics into focus and to challenge the accuracy of the story.

The Healing Relationship

From Carl Rogers we have learned the value of relating to patients in a nonpossessive, accepting way and expressing our caring by providing accurate empathy.[36] The accepting practitioner creates a safe environment that facilitates the exploration of various possibilities for change.

Empathic understanding is communicated to the patient through techniques of active and accurate listening. This is demonstrated by first listening to the story without interrupting for one or two minutes and then paraphrasing, summarizing, reflecting feelings, and responding authentically. According to Rogers, however, these techniques are relatively unimportant except as a channel for communicating positive regard and accurate empathy.[36] Sometimes, it takes a while for the patient to receive the communication. Repeated visits to a primary care practitioner create the perfect medium to allow the message to sink in.

Behavioral Therapies

The evolution of behavioral therapies since Bandura[37] first conceptualized psychotherapy as a learning process in the early 1960s has been phenomenal. In a review of 252 empirical studies of psychotherapy in the three decades from 1967–1968 to 1987–1988, H. Omer and R. Dar[38] document the striking evolution away from theory-guided research to pragmatic, clinically oriented research. However, empirical studies of psychotherapy continue to present formidable obstacles.[39]

The popularity of behavioral approaches to therapy can be attributed to their utility in helping patients find solutions for their problems in living. Relaxation, desensitization, visualization, assertiveness training, and biofeedback all stem from behaviorism in that patients practice and learn new ways to manage themselves, their anxiety, and their behavior. Research has repeatedly demonstrated that thinking is a behavior that can be modified and that modes of thinking affect the origin, maintenance, and change process related to various human problems.[40] People are often not aware that how they think about a situation directly influences how they feel about it. Albert Ellis points out that when we think about our goals, even the process of planning steps that we can take to further these goals results in positive feelings.[41]

Ellis continues to underscore the importance of identifying the rigid, dogmatic, and powerful demands and commands that constitute the irrational beliefs most of us hold regarding the way the world is supposed to be. He points out that it is important to dispute statements such as "It's awful" (meaning totally bad or more than bad!) or "I can't bear it" (meaning survive or be happy at all!).[40] Cognitive behavioral therapy has many variations and is used for many types of psychiatric disorders. A.T. Beck and J.D. Young[42] have very successfully used these techniques to help severely depressed persons counter the negative thoughts and evaluations of self, others, and circumstances that trigger and maintain depressive syndromes. Schema-focused therapy[43] incorporates cognitive, experiential, interpersonal, and behavioral techniques for working with patients with personality disorders and other difficult chronic syndromes. D.H. Barlow[44] combines cognitive techniques with various forms of relaxation training in the treatment of panic and other anxiety disorders. These techniques are powerful, especially when promoted by a primary care practitioner.

Relaxation Training

It is not difficult to teach patients techniques to help them relax. It also does not take a great deal of time. These techniques can be learned easily during a 15-minute visit. It does, however, require the patient to practice the techniques daily, for periods of perhaps 10 minutes, for at least two weeks. Practitioners must explain to patients that the experience of anxiety or stress is mutually exclusive with relaxation. When stressed, patients will take shallow and rapid breaths, tense their muscles, and experience racing, negative thoughts. To physically control stress and anxiety, patients are instructed to focus on their breathing, exhaling completely while trying to push their stomachs into their spines. When they inhale they will fill their lungs all the way to their diaphragms. This is called "belly breathing." It results in a relaxation response. It focuses patients' attention on their breathing, puts them in control of this normally automatic behavior, and is a powerful antidote to stress. Ideally, patients will do this for a few minutes several times each day, but it can be used as needed during periods of stress. As previously stated, this type of breathing does require a certain amount of practice to become comfortable and ultimately automatic.

Patients can also be instructed to intentionally relax their muscles. It is good to start by having patients alternately tense and relax specific muscle groups in order to help them recognize the difference between tension and relaxation. They can focus on hands, arms, and shoulders; then the face and neck; followed by feet, legs, and buttocks; and finally chest and abdomen. After all muscle groups have been completely relaxed, patients will enjoy relief of pain and stress. Once they have learned to control their breathing and relax their muscles, patients can also be instructed to repeat positive thoughts to themselves. After a little more practice, they can learn to visualize and create mental representations of healing experiences. These techniques can be used to countermand a variety of symptoms from anxiety, headaches, and general tension to chronic pain. They can be thought of as "behavioral aspirin," powerful therapeutic interventions with no negative side effects. The techniques empower patients and give them positive choices. The instructions can be reinforced by patient education handouts or recommending self-help books, some of which are listed in Appendix B, but the power of the intervention derives from being taught and monitored by primary care practitioners and the stated assurance about its efficacy.

Narrative Therapy

A new therapy that has gained recognition in the last decade is narrative therapy.[45] Michael White, an Australian practitioner, built on the notion that all our knowledge of the world is carried through mental maps of external reality. Since no map includes every detail of the territory, events that do not make it onto the map do not exist in that map's world of meaning. White saw that "a story is map that extends through time."[45] This postmodern, narrative, social constructionist world view offers useful ideas about how power, knowledge, and "truth" are negotiated in families and larger cultures. The basic theses of "postmodernism," or the social constructionist viewpoint, include the following:

1. Realities are socially constructed.
2. Realities are constituted through language.
3. Realities are organized and maintained through narrative.
4. There are no essential truths.

Michael White introduced "relative influence questioning" as a way to separate patients from their problems and help them to invent more positive stories. Patients are asked to map the influence of a particular problem on their lives and their relationships and then to map their influence on the life of the problem. Rather than being the problem, people have relationships with the problem. They are then invited to speculate about changing the future. What would their life be like if they did not have this problem? Would this be a preferred experience? How would they act? How would they feel? Was there a time in the past when they felt that way? What did they do differently at the time? Then they are asked to link the two episodes. This is followed by questions that extend the story into the future. Narrative therapists ask questions to generate experiences rather than to gather information. White suggests that when we ask questions, we are generating possible versions of a life. Experience is colored and shaped by the meaning people give it. Whether people attend to the experience is related to the stories people are living. Narrative therapy makes a shift from gathering information to generating experience. We contend that questions intentionally asked by primary care practitioners can be powerful therapeutic interventions. Questions posed do not necessarily have to be answered during a session but can be left as unfinished business for the patient to consider.

White distinguishes five specific kinds of questions. "*Deconstruction questions*" unpack the story and help people to see different perspectives. They are invited to distinguish particular beliefs, practices, feelings, and attitudes. Practitioners might ask about history, context, effects or results, interrelationships, and tactics or strategies. "*Opening space questions*" inquire about unique outcomes. They probe hypothetical experiences and different contexts and time frames; for example, "In what situations do you have a different reaction?" "*Preference questions*" look at whether the patient would be better or worse off without the problem. "*Story development questions*" invite people to relate the process and details of an experience and to connect it to a time frame, a particular context, and other people; and "*meaning questions*" explore patients' motivations, hopes, goals, values, and beliefs. Story development and meaning questions help in story reconstruction. These techniques are not only practical but also highly effective and can be used to explore patients' stories about their health and disease as well as social functioning.

Expecting Patient Follow-Through

According to William Glasser, M.D., patients develop symptoms and engage in irresponsible behavior because they are not controlling their lives and they choose not to feel the painful emotions triggered by the situation.[46] Often, these painful emotions are converted to physical pain in various parts of the body. Glasser considers what is labeled as mental illness, regardless of the causation, to be the hundreds of ways people choose to behave when they are unable to satisfy their innate needs for love and power to the extent they want. When patients do not feel worthwhile to themselves and others (competent) or loved (connected), they need the warmth, kindness, and strength of a practitioner who will support them while at the same time holding them responsible for changing their behavior. Using Glasser's approach, the practitioner acts as a coach, encouraging the patient to focus on current behavior, evaluate that behavior, and plan alternate (more constructive) behavior. The crux of reality therapy is that the patient is expected to take responsibility for follow-through. No excuses are accepted. If a plan is reasonable, there are no excuses. At the same time, there is no punishment. There is consistent insistence that commitments be honored. Patients become aware that there are consequences in real life for poor choices and failure to carry out commitments. The therapeutic relationship, however, remains one of respect, caring, and involvement through mutual setting of reasonable expectations and monitoring of results. These interventions combine the best of theory and pragmatic application, and they really work.

DETERMINING LEVELS OF INVOLVEMENT IN PRACTICE: PLISSIT

Having outlined key mechanisms that create the need for counseling and the critical elements of the therapeutic encounter, we would like to specify exactly how this understanding can be translated into primary care practice.

Any encounter that inspires the patient's hopes for improvement, be it one visit or several, is therapeutic. For the primary care practitioner, however, it is useful to have a protocol to guide the level of intervention. A mechanistic but practical and effective hierarchical system was first introduced by J.S. Annon in the context of sex therapy.[47] This four-step process triggered by the acronym "PLISSIT" is easily remembered and simple to apply.

In a potentially therapeutic situation, where the patient is concerned with certain reactions to a particular situation, the levels of intervention go from permission giving, to offering limited information, to specific suggestions, to a contract for intensive therapy.

P Stands for Permission

Regardless of what else transpires in the therapeutic session, it is always appropriate to give patients permission to feel what they feel. This simple intervention does more to restore patients' equilibrium than almost anything else the practitioner can do. When patients become aware that the world or other people are not as they want them to be or that they are not handling situations as well as they want to, they feel bad. When the practitioner reassures the patient the reaction that is being experienced is normal under the circumstances, the patient feels better. The patient recognizes that it is O.K. to be depressed and does not have to be depressed about being depressed. The patient may have lost his temper and yelled at his wife. The practitioner assures him it is O.K. to get angry, especially when one is under stress. Under the circumstances, that can happen. However, the patient needs to let his wife know that he is sorry. It is important to give people permission to feel the way they feel, because if they could feel any other way, at that particular time, they would. The practitioner's understanding and acceptance make the patient feel more comfortable with the emotional state being experienced.

LI Stands for Limited Information

The second level of intervention is to provide a small amount of essential information that explains the emotional state being experienced. This helps patients set realistic expectations for themselves and others. For example, a patient in a situation of crisis is told that in general, when people experience great amounts of stress, they react by feeling overwhelmed, confused, and less capable of making decisions or solving problems; have trouble sleeping; and so on. This normalization helps get the patient off *tilt*. The patient feels as though under the circumstances the reaction is appropriate after all. Information processing is a high-order coping skill. By offering accurate and pertinent information, in small enough amounts for the patient to assimilate, the practitioner is leading to the patient's strength.

SS Stands for Specific Suggestions

Specific suggestions can be given to the patient to examine options, answer specific questions, talk to friends, get into a self-help group, take time out, keep a journal, or employ any other specific strategy that helps to engage the patient's healthy functioning self and promote constructive coping behavior. These suggestions must be tailored to fit into the patient's current lifestyle and not present one more overwhelming demand. Often it is useful to ask the patient, "What one thing could you do that would make you feel a little better?" or "What can you do to get more information before you make that important decision?" The practitioner's interest and confidence that the patient is competent and in control foster this behavior in the patient.

IT Stands for Intensive Therapy

Intensive therapy as it applies to the primary care setting implies that the practitioner makes a commitment to work with the patient over time. Appointments are scheduled, and the practitioner contracts to offer support for the patient for a specific time in order to resolve a particular life problem. By engaging in a therapeutic contract with the patient, all five criteria specified in the section on common psychotherapeutic elements are satisfied. Positive expectations that help is forthcoming are instigated. A therapeutic relationship is established. The patient receives an external perspective on the problem. Corrective experiences are encouraged, and the patient is given the opportunity to test reality repeatedly. The practitioner connects with the patient and helps to further his or her sense of competency.

SUMMARY

Practical therapeutic interventions treat emotional, behavioral, personality, or psychiatric disorders, primarily through communication with the patient. Psychotherapy is the process of helping patients edit their "stories." Therapeutic goals are generic (making patients feel better and less overwhelmed) and specific (making patients feel competent and connected to others).

Supportive therapy focuses on the patient's strength, whereas exploratory therapy traces the etiology of feelings. It is more important to help patients change their reactions than to understand their source. Common elements among psychotherapeutic techniques include (1) the expectation of receiving help, (2) participation in a therapeutic relationship, (3) obtaining an external perspective on problems, (4) the encouragement of corrective experiences, and (5) the opportunity to test reality repeatedly.

Language is used to record and classify our perceptual experience of the world. Through processes of generalization, deletion, and distortion, people build impoverished "maps," or models of the world, which then limit their perceived options. The therapeutic process challenges these generalizations, deletions, and distortions in order to create a richer representation of possibilities. There is a growing body of research that empirically connects people's explanations of why something happened to their subsequent emotional and physical state. People's sense of self-efficacy is directly related to outcomes. In general, people are simpler than insight schools give them credit for but more complex than behavioral models suggest. Carl Rogers's contribution relates to the value of accurate empathy and nonpossessive caring in a therapeutic relationship. Behavior therapies underscore the importance of human learning in the process of modifying behavior. Cognitive therapy is based on modifying "irrational" beliefs that affect how people react to situations. The word "yet" is a powerful therapeutic tool. It is not difficult to teach patients techniques of belly breathing and muscle relaxation to manage stress and anxiety. It also does not take a great deal of time. Narrative therapy uses focused questions to help the patient reconstruct reality. Through the creation of a warm and understanding relationship, a practitioner encourages patients to accept responsibility for their behavior.

The acronym "PLISSIT" can be used to structure levels of intervention, from simple permission giving, to offering limited information, making specific suggestions, or entering into a contract for intensive therapy.

REFERENCES

1. Frank, J.D. *Persuasion and Healing*, rev. ed. Baltimore: Johns Hopkins, 1973.
2. Welwood, J. *Journey of the Heart: Intimate Relationship and the Path of Love*. New York: Harper Collins, 1990, p. 25.
3. Leichsenring, F. Comparative effects of short-term psychodynamic psychotherapy and cognitive-behavioral therapy in depression: A meta-analytic approach. *Clinical Psychology Review*, 2001, *21*, 401–419.
4. Seligman, M. The effectiveness of psychotherapy: The Consumer Reports study. *American Psychologist*, 1995, *50*, 965–974.
5. Tylee, A. Depression in the community: Physician and patient perspective. *Journal of Clinical Psychiatry*, 1999, *60*(suppl. 7), 12–16.
6. Maier, W., & Falkai, P. The epidemiology of comorbidity between depression, anxiety disorders and somatic diseases. *International Clinical Psychopharmacology*, 1999, *14*(suppl. 2), S1–6.
7. Melartin, T., & Isometsae, E. Psychiatric comorbidity of major depressive disorder—a review. *Psychiatria Fennica*, 2000, *31*, 87–100.
8. Rodin, J. *Aging and health: Effects of the sense of control*. Science, 1986, *233*, 1271–1275.
9. Schaubroeck, J., Jones, J.R., & Xie, J.L. Individual differences in utilizing control to cope with job demands: Effects on susceptibility to infectious disease. *Journal of Applied Psychology*, 2001, *86*(2), 265–278.
10. Miller, G.E., & Cohen, S. Psychological interventions and the immune system: A meta-analytic review and critique. *Health Psychology*, 2001, *20*, 47–63.
11. Kiecolt-Glasser, J.K., & Glaser, R. Psychosocial moderators of immune function. *Annals of Behavioral Medicine*, 1987, *9*, 16–20.
12. Frank, J.D. Therapeutic components. In Myers, J.M. (ed.) *Cures by Psychotherapy: What Effects Change?* New York: Praeger, 1984.
13. Watzlawick, P., Weakland, J.H., & Fisch, R. *Change: Principles of Problem Formation and Problem Resolution*. New York: W.W. Norton & Co., 1974.

14. Goldfried, M.R. Rapproachment of psychotherapies. *Journal of Humanistic Psychology*, 1983, *23*, 97–107.
15. Frank, J.D. Psychotherapy: The restoration of morale. *American Journal of Psychiatry*, 1974, *131*, 271–274.
16. de Figueiredo, J.M., & Frank, J.D. Subjective incompetence, the clinical hallmark of demoralization. *Comprehensive Psychiatry*, 1982, *23*, 253–263.
17. Bandler, R., & Grinder, J. *The Structure of Magic. I. A Book About Language and Therapy.* Palo Alto, Calif.: Science and Behavior Books, 1975.
18. Seligman, M.E.P. Learned helplessness. *Annual Review of Medicine*, 1972, *23*, 407–412.
19. Peterson, C., & Seligman, M.E.P. Casual explanations as a risk factor for depression: Theory and evidence. *Psychological Review*, 1984, *91*, 347–374.
20. Peterson, C., & Seligman, M.E.P. Explanatory style and illness. *Journal of Personality*, 1987, *55*, 237–265.
21. Seligman, M.E.P. *Helplessness: On Depression, Development, and Death.* San Francisco: Freeman, 1975.
22. van Doorn, C. A qualitative approach to studying health optimism, realism, and pessimism. *Research on Aging*, 1999, *21*, 440–457.
23. Kamen, L.P., & Seligman, M.E.P. Explanatory style and health. *Current Psychological Research and Reviews*, 1987, *6*, 207–218.
24. Peterson, C., Seligman, M.E.P., & Vaillant, G.E. Pessimistic explanatory style is a risk factor for physical illness: A thirty-five year longitudinal study. *Journal of Personality and Social Psychology*, 1988, *55*, 23–27.
25. Kamen-Siegel, L., Rodin, J., Seligman, M.E.P., & Dwyer, J. Explanatory style and cell-mediated immunity in elderly men and women. *Health Psychology*, 1991, *10*(4), 229–235.
26. Burns, M.O., & Seligman, M.E.P. Explanatory style across the life-span: Evidence for stability over fifty-two years. *Journal of Personality and Social Psychology*, 1989, *56*, 471–477.
27. Bandura, A. Self-efficacy: Toward a unifying theory of behavioral change. *Psychological Review*, 1977, *84*(2), 191–215.
28. Wigal, J.K., Creer, T.L., & Kotses, H. The COPD Self-Efficacy Scale. *Chest*, 1991, *99*(5), 1193–1196.
29. Fitzgerald, S.T., Becker, D.M., Celkentano, D.D., Swank, R., & Brinker, J. Return to work after percutaneous transluminal coronary angioplasty. *American Journal of Cardiology*, 1989, *64*, 1108–1112.
30. Arnstein, P. The mediation of disability by self-efficacy in different samples of chronic pain patients. *Disability & Rehabilitation: An International Multidisciplinary Journal*, 2000, *22*(17), 794–801.
31. Waldrop, D., Lightsey, O.R., Ethington, C.A., Woemmel, C.A., & Coke, A.L. Self-efficacy, optimism, health competence, and recovery from orthopedic surgery. *Journal of Counseling Psychology*, 2001, *48*(2), 233–238.
32. Cunningham, A.J., Lockwood, G.A., & Cunningham, J.A. A relationship between perceived self-efficacy and quality of life in cancer patients. *Patient Education and Counseling*, 1991, *17*(1), 71–78.
33. Sullivan, M., LaCroix, A.Z., Russo, J., & Katon, W.J. Self-efficacy and self-reported functional status in coronary heart disease: A six-month prospective study. *Psychosomatic Medicine*, 1998, *60*(4), 473–478.
34. Bandura, A. Recycling misconceptions of perceived self-efficacy. *Cognitive Therapy & Research*, 1984, *8*, 231–255.
35. Taylor, S.E., Kemeny, M.E., Reed, G.M., Bower, J.E., & Gruenewald, T.L. Psychological resources, positive illusions and health. *American Psychologist*, 2000, *55*(1), 99–109.
36. Rogers, C. The necessary and sufficient conditions of therapeutic personality change. *Journal of Consulting Psychology*, 1957, *21*, 95–103.
37. Bandura, A. Psychotherapy as a learning process. *Psychological Bulletin*, 1961, *58*, 143–159.
38. Omer, H., & Dar, R. Changing trends in three decades of psychotherapy research: The flight from theory into pragmatics. *Journal of Consulting & Clinical Psychology*, 1992, *60*, 88–93.
39. Henry, W.P. Science, politics and the politics of science: The use and misuse of empirically validated treatment research. *Psychotherapy Research*, 1998, *8*, 126–140.
40. Ellis, A. The revised ABC's of rational-emotive therapy (RET). *Journal of Rational-Emotive & Cognitive-Behavior Therapy*, 1991, *9*, 139–172.
41. Ellis. p. 144.
42. Beck, A.T., & Young, J.E. Depression. In Barlow, D.H. (ed.) *Clinical Handbook of Psychological Disorders.* New York: Guilford Press, 1985, pp. 206–244.
43. Young, J.D. *Cognitive Therapy for Personality Disorders: A Schema-Focused Approach*, 3rd ed. Sarasota, Fla.: Professional Resource Press, 1999.
44. Barlow, D.H. Long-term outcome for patients with panic disorder treated with cognitive-behavioral therapy. *Journal of Clinical Psychiatry*, 1990, *51*(suppl. A), 17–23.

45. Freedan, J., & Combs, G. *Narrative Therapy: The Social Construction of Preferred Realities*. New York: W.W. Norton & Co., 1996.
46. Glasser, W. *Reality Therapy in Action*. New York: Harper Collins, 2000.
47. Annon, J.S. *Behavioral Treatment of Sexual Problems: Brief Therapy*. New York: Harper & Row, 1976.

CHAPTER 5

Differences in Approach Between Primary Care Practitioners and Psychiatrists

Obviously there are major differences in both process and outcome between therapeutic interventions that are provided by primary care practitioners and traditional treatment by psychiatrists or other mental health professionals. Collaborative mental health care, ideally with counselors actually located within the primary care setting, is a more recent option.[1,2] Studies of psychosocial treatments in primary care provide support for the effectiveness of this type of intervention.[3,4] We would like to explore from several angles differences between counseling that is provided in the primary care setting and services that are either "carved out" or obtained by referrals to mental health specialists. We are primarily interested in the effect of the practitioner's direct interventions. After looking at patient expectations and reactions, we will examine key aspects of the doctor-patient relationship, delineate the practitioner's investment in the patient's problems, and lastly, recommend some specific therapeutic approaches that are particularly suited to the therapeutic structure of primary care.

There is an old story about a secretary who went to work for a psychiatrist. After only a few short weeks, she resigned. When asked why she quit the job, she reported to her friends, "I just couldn't win. He was always analyzing everything I did. If I got to work late, he said it was because I was hostile. When I got to work early, he wondered why I was anxious. Those days I got to work on time, he accused me of being compulsive."

Psychiatrists deal with a selected sample of humanity and learn what they know about people through interaction with their patients.[5] Primary care practitioners see a different spectrum of patients presenting with undifferentiated problems. Psychiatrists are trained to look for psychopathological conditions and to describe and classify the observed phenomena according to the appropriate category in the American Psychiatric Association's *Diagnostic and Statistical Manual of Mental Disorders*, 4th ed., text revision (DSM-IV-TR).[6] Devising a coherent theoretical explanation for the etiology of the symptom is usually part of the diagnostic process. Although in psychiatry the process of making a diagnosis is considered to be part of the treatment,[5] this activity often intimidates patients who are most commonly referred because of stress or relationship problems.[4]

Regardless of other presenting problems, we believe it is part of the primary care practitioner's task to look for and treat psychological distress experienced by patients. If the emotional component is left untreated, patients are apt to attempt to relieve their suffering by repeated and often inappropriate use of medical services.[7] However, psychosocial information should be gathered in a therapeutic manner, providing support rather than generating additional stress for the patient.

PATIENT FACTORS

When a practitioner initiates a psychiatric referral, whether to a mental health center or to an individual practitioner, an acknowledgment of the appropriateness of the referral is generally followed by a request to have the patient personally call to set up the initial appointment. It is accepted practice to consider the patient's request for help as the first step in the therapeutic process, but this requires the patient's cooperation.

Referrals Are Often Not Completed

Patients are often reluctant to admit that they need psychiatric treatment.[8] The idea of defining themselves as mental patients is an impediment to seeking help. A study of utilization data from the Civilian Health and Medical Program of the Uniformed Services (CHAMPUS) showed that from 1982 to 1987, visits for outpatient behavioral health treatment increased by 35%, but psychiatrists' share of that market dropped from 36% to less than 22%, while treatment by primary care practitioners doubled.[9] Even when referrals are made, patients often do not follow through.[10] Studies show that somewhere between 15% and 75% of patients who are referred for psychotherapy fail to keep initial appointments.[11,12] Those patients who are most resistant to completing referrals also make more medical visits, generally presenting with difficult-to-explain somatic symptoms.[13] Even when referral is successful, 30% to 60% of psychiatric patients in outpatient clinics drop out after only two to five sessions for a variety of reasons.[14,15] The reported attrition rate for private psychiatrists is almost as high.[16] There is some evidence that even a single session of psychotherapy can be very effective, because of the ego-strengthening function implied in such brief treatment.[17] However, when patients are referred and it is not their idea, not only is the dropout rate high, but also, according to a study by C.L. Bowden and his colleagues,[18] about half of the patients dropping out feel worse than when starting treatment.

Referrals Carry a Price Tag

Every employment application asks whether you have been treated for a mental or emotional disorder. Once treatment by a psychiatrist or other mental health professional has been obtained, patients have two choices: to lie about their medical history or to identify themselves as mental patients. Mental patients are often seen as people who have been or are suffering from a disorder that carries a social stigma. Politicians whose histories reveal treatment for depression or other emotional conditions frequently become unacceptable to the public. It is not having been depressed that marks the flawed candidate; it is a "record" of having been diagnosed and treated for an affective disorder, a mental disease. Although in some social circles, comparing notes about what one's analyst has to say may be an accepted cocktail party sport, many middle- and lower-class patients are intimidated by the prospect of a psychiatric consultation.

Thomas Szasz[19] is perhaps the best known critic of psychiatric labeling, but others have noted that psychiatric labeling can be used in pejorative ways as a form of social coercion.[19-21] Certainly, when treatment is proposed before the patient has recognized the need, this can be initially deflating to the patient's already fragile self-esteem. The resulting damage to the sense of self-worth must then be restored before any positive therapeutic effect can take place.

PROVIDING SERVICES IN THE PRIMARY CARE SETTING

It is not our intention to discount the value of psychiatry or psychotherapy as generally practiced. We are talking about treating a different patient population. Psychiatrists are specialists trained to treat people who are seriously ill. They may well be wasting their talents treating those who are less disturbed. Not every case of chest pain warrants referral to a cardiologist. Even when referral is indicated, many patients experience serious impediments to receiving psychiatric treatment. Some of these obstacles are financial, some are logistical, and some have to do with the patient's reluctance to pursue treatment.[22] Better outcomes can be expected when mental health services are directly integrated into primary care.[23] In our view, some very important and effective therapeutic interventions can be made directly by primary care practitioners. Further, these interventions are different in several respects from those generally employed by psychiatrists. Let us look at some of these differences.

Treatment of Symptoms Without Psychiatric Labeling

The first major difference is that the primary care practitioner can treat the patient's emotional reaction to whatever environmental stress is being experienced without labeling the patient as a mental patient. The patient receives the help that is asked for (relief of symptoms) and does not have to deal with the idea of seeing a "shrink." Actually, it has been our experience that after working with the primary care practitioner on the emotional overlay attached to various physical problems, patients will often request a referral to a mental health practitioner in order to extend their work of self-exploration. One of the most beneficial aspects of the therapeutic relationship with the primary care practitioner may be to prepare the patient for needed in-depth psychological treatment.[24] When patients start to experience the benefits that result from increased levels of personal awareness and control, they often overcome the reluctance to engage in psychiatric treatment. However, for many patients the timely intervention by the practitioner restores normal functioning or even improves normal functioning to such an extent that the need for further treatment is precluded.

Small Doses of Therapy at a Time

The second major difference between therapeutic interventions provided by the primary care practitioner and traditional psychiatric treatment is that the patient receives small doses of psychotherapy as a part of the regular medical visit. Every part of the interaction with the practitioner is potentially therapeutic. We have gone to great lengths to point out the amount of social power that is attributed to practitioners. Because of this power, the personal exchanges, both verbal and nonverbal, that occur during the normal office visit can have tremendous impact on the patient. Since each of us has an assumptive map, a mental representation of ourselves and our world based on personal history as we have recorded it (our story), our perception of ourselves can be influenced by how we see ourselves treated by significant others with whom we come in contact.[25-27] If our story line has been that we are not at all important and that no one cares about us and then, over time, we are repeatedly treated well by an important person, after some initial discounting and disbelief we may change our assumptive map and edit our story. As the weight of evidence countering our preconceived notions of ourselves increases, we are able to make a change in our self-image. It may actually take the form of a paradigm shift (as explained in Chapter 1).

Small repeated doses of therapeutic messages may actually be more effective, in terms of being heard, believed, and integrated, than a large dose at any one time, which may be more difficult to swallow and to assimilate. People learn by repetition over a period of time but only when it is psychologically safe for them to do so and when they are ready to learn.

The Patient Does Not Feel Rejected

The third major factor to be considered in providing psychological treatment personally rather than making a referral, even when appropriate, is that often the patient may interpret the referral as rejection. If the patient feels comfortable with and trusts the practitioner, there is a natural reluctance to start over with someone new. Being referred may also play into the self-deprecating pathological view of the patient. When a patient's self-esteem is low and the practitioner responds by pushing the patient away, sending the patient to see someone else, this may confirm the patient's view that "no one can or wants to help." The patient may feel that there is little use in even trying. In contrast, the practitioner's commitment to helping the patient is interpreted as an indication that the situation may be far less serious than the patient has assumed and that the patient is more worthy of help. Naturally, there will be times that a referral must be made because the practitioner feels overwhelmed. We will discuss this in a subsequent section.

The Body and the Mind Are Not Separated

Especially in the case of psychosomatic illness, rather than exploring all the organic elements before trying to convince the patient that psychological treatment is indicated and possibly making the patient feel inadequate and raising resistance, we treat physical and psychological components of the problem concurrently, which may, over time, convince the patient of the connection. This moves the patient in a positive direction toward addressing the underlying problem. Writing in the *New England Journal of Medicine* about functional gastrointestinal disorders, J.E. Lennard-Jones pointed out the importance of making the psychosocial history part of the initial inquiry "because a sudden interest in possible psychological factors after investigations have given normal results can arouse hostility in the patient."[28] Patients with psychosomatic problems who are referred to psychiatrists after a full exploration of their somatic complaints are notorious for seeking further medical opinions and being refractory to psychiatric treatment.[29,30] In addition, the focus on purely organic problems is not necessarily benign. Harrington has pointed out that practitioners often unwittingly precipitate or perpetuate patients' emotional illness. "Every psychiatrist sees patients who have been in the hands of three or four different specialists, all of whom are said to have told the patient something different. Such patients are hard to treat because they have lost faith."[31]

PRACTITIONER-PATIENT RELATIONSHIP

There are several distinct differences in the relationship between a patient and a primary care practitioner and that with a psychiatrist. The relationship with the primary care practitioner has continuity over time and is predicated on receiving whatever care is necessary to keep the patient healthy and functioning at optimum levels. Patients' emotional responses are a logical concomitant of their physical condition and can be treated as such. In contrast, a relationship with a psychiatrist is specifically focused on eradicating some mental aberration or personality defect that is interfering with the patient's ability to function. This interference must be serious enough to overcome the patient's resistance to psychiatric treatment.

The Effects of the Psychiatric Evaluation Process

The initial psychiatric interview is structured to establish rapport with the patient while determining the etiology and extent of the patient's psychopathological condition. The psychiatrist will draw inferences from the behavior of the patient toward the interviewer. Many people, not only psychiatric patients, feel very uncomfortable when they know that they are being analyzed and evaluated, especially by an expert. As a result, they may become defensive. When patients share information about various aspects of their functioning with the primary care practitioner, they may feel much more comfortable about disclosing personal information. This is especially true when the information is elicited over a series of visits.

Knowledge of the Family

The primary care practitioner is often acquainted with various members of the patient's family. If the practitioner already knows the circumstances of a patient's family constellation and has had personal contact with the cast of characters involved, it becomes easier to empathize with the patient's experience. "Yes, I know Mary can be difficult to deal with. What can you do to make her feel more secure?" can be a powerful intervention, coming from someone who has had dealings with Mary. The patient already trusts the practitioner, whereas the psychiatrist is an unknown individual who is suspect simply because of being cast in the role of psychiatrist, that is, evaluator and analyst.

The Gift of Caring

Perhaps the most crucial difference in the character of the primary care practitioner-patient relationship as opposed to the psychiatrist-patient relationship is that in the former whatever psychological support is received is seen as a bonus. Although it may not always be intuitively obvious, there is a difference between psychological support that is received and that which is given. Unfortunately, when on *tilt*, we are often unreceptive to positive messages that are directed at us. It is necessary to be open to hearing supportive statements. If self-esteem is exceedingly low, being told by another that we are perfectly capable and will be O.K. is interpreted as false reassurance and a further confirmation that no one understands how dreadful we feel and how awful everything is.

A patient seeks psychiatric treatment in order to feel better. The patient expects the psychiatrist to be helpful and provide support. Instead, the psychiatrist may stress the patient in order to uncover pathological conditions and obtain pertinent information to make an accurate diagnosis before prescribing pharmacological treatment. A practitioner is expected to provide medical diagnosis and treatment. Increasingly, studies are documenting the importance of practitioners also providing for the socioemotional needs of patients with outcomes related not only to patient satisfaction but also to patients' subsequent health.[32-35]

Williard Gaylin, in his insightful book *Caring*,[36] discusses the importance of finding outlets to express the caring impulse that is biologically programmed into the human species. He makes the following point that clarifies the impact of the practitioner's interest in the psychological adjustment of the patient:

> . . . We are generally touched by behavior that does more for us than we might have expected, (and) we are hurt by behavior that does less for us than we feel we have a right to expect. It is my feeling that in most senses of the usage, being touched and feeling hurt are polar phenomena. I am touched by your solicitude and hurt by your lack of solicitude; touched by the fact that despite a limited acquaintance, you remembered my birthday; hurt by the fact that even though you are my spouse, you had forgotten. If being touched is preeminently visualized in terms of the delighted and somewhat unexpected caring attitude of an individual, feeling hurt is the absence of such an attitude where we feel entitled to it and where we have every reason to expect it. In that sense we can see where we are more likely to be hurt by those who are close to us and touched by casual friends. In both cases there is an unexpected and unwarranted quality. Those who know us slightly honor us with their affection or attention, as those who know us well abuse us by failing to show that they care. To feel hurt occurs with a failure in caring. This, then, represents our vulnerability through attachments, or need to feel cared for.[37]

If the psychiatrist fails to give the expected support or appears to be cold and distant, the patient feels hurt. On the other hand, the practitioner's interest in the psychological aspect of the patient's condition is received as a gift of caring. The patient is generally touched. This touch is healing. The bonus for the practitioner is that the patient responds positively to the clinician, increasing compliance and satisfaction for both parties.

ADOPTING A HOLISTIC VIEW OF THE PATIENT

The primary care practitioner has the special opportunity and responsibility to relate to the patient not from solely a physiological or a psychological perspective. Our approach to the patient is based on the assumption that the basic biological unit reacting to demands from the environment encompasses the body, mind, and spirit in dynamic interaction. This is hardly a revolutionary idea. More than 40 years ago, John Nemiah, a noted professor of psychiatry at Harvard Medical School, wrote as follows:

> The practitioner who limits himself, whether it be to the confines of physiology or psychology, does so to the detriment of his patient. The art and practice of medicine require on the part of the doctor an awareness that human life is a process lived in a constantly changing world which requires, for survival, a constantly adaptive response . . . . Rational treatment is based on helping the patient return to health by combating the forces upsetting the balance—whether physiological or psychological.[38]

It is the role of the primary care practitioner to understand that the mind and body together constitute the complete unit of the individual who is integrally influenced by stimuli from the external and internal environments while maintaining a particular spiritual orientation. By connecting with the patient psychologically while at the same time "laying on hands" in the process of examining the body, the practitioner has the unique power to help the patient correct whatever disturbance in homeostasis has precipitated the visit to the doctor.

The psychiatrist, on the other hand, is more narrowly focused on the psychodynamics of the personality. By putting emphasis largely on mind instead of body, the reverse split achieves no more productive result than looking for pathological conditions only in tissues and organs. The tendency to specialize fragments care for the person. It may well be that fragmentation in the fabric of our society, or the structure of the patient's family or work situation, is precipitating the illness in the first place. The changing model of "health care" (see Chapter 1) requires that the body, mind, and spirit be integrated, since a demoralized patient can maintain neither physical nor mental health.

Thus the major difference in approach is that the primary care practitioner, in contrast to the mental health specialist, helps the patient make a more comfortable adaptation to the existing environment, without getting into the specific technicalities of the patient's personality structure, specific defense mechanisms, or even family dynamics, since these are difficult to change (except in a crisis). Instead, the practitioner focuses on the reaction that the person is experiencing to perceived stress from the environment. This reaction may be anxiety, depression, or any number of physical complaints. By providing support and focusing the patient on constructive action, the practitioner helps to enhance the patient's self-esteem and enables the patient to function at a more productive level.

THE PRACTITIONER'S VIEW OF THE PROBLEM

Perhaps the most important factor to keep in mind when doing counseling in the 15-minute framework is that the problem belongs to the patient. The process of medical education predisposes the practitioner to take on and solve problems. The first step in problem solving is to accurately define the problem. In this case the problem must be defined as the patient's reaction. The practitioner cannot afford to get intimately involved in the details of the situation or understand the exact etiology or even the specific effect of the circumstances on all the people involved. The practitioner is not responsible for solving the patient's problem. Rather, the practitioner's responsibility is limited to supporting the patient so that the patient can identify the specific problem that may be underlying the experienced stress, making the patient aware that this problem is contributing to the feelings of illness that he or she is experiencing, and encouraging the patient to explore potential solutions for the problem, as in the following example:

Mrs. K., a 30-year-old Asian mother of a three-month-old boy, is in the office for the third time in two weeks. She is complaining about feeling tired all the time, with headaches and some dizziness. She says that her body feels strange. On previous visits it has been determined that she is not anemic. Mrs. K. is delighted with her baby and reports that her husband is very supportive and concerned and that her mother is living with them and helping to care for the child. As he leaves the room after an uneventful exam, the practitioner wonders what is really going on. He speculates whether having her mom there is making the patient feel competitive for the baby's attention. Perhaps the lifestyle change triggered by the birth is causing a conflict. Armed with specific theories, the doctor reenters the exam room. "Mrs. K., I really am sorry that you feel so bad. I found nothing during my exam to cause me any concern. Still, something is causing your symptoms. What do you think it might be?"

At first, the patient looks at him blankly and says nothing. The practitioner inquires, "What is going on in your life?" Hesitantly, the patient discloses that her mother is planning to return to Hong Kong and leave her to manage the baby alone. The practitioner asks how she feels about that. She admits that she is afraid to function independently, does not want to be cut off from her mom and the outside world, and feels inadequate to care for her son. The doctor explains how anxiety can produce physical symptoms. He then focuses on supporting the patient, accepting her feelings, and asking her to think about what skills she must learn while her mother is still there. Another appointment is made. His plan is to enhance her sense of self-efficacy (see Chapter 4) in an effort to convince her that she is capable of performing as a mother. He will motivate her by focusing on how important this is to her and how she can gain the necessary skill and confidence. He will also continue to be there for her and provide support and advice.

When the practitioner communicates the expectation that the patient, having identified the problem, will find some constructive resolution, a positive message is conveyed. The patient is empowered. The practitioner agrees to be part of the process, support initiatives, and make suggestions for strategies that can be employed, but it is clear to both parties that the patient has the responsibility to deal with the problem (which, by definition, is expected to yield to resolution).

Focus on the Present

Our approach, which focuses almost exclusively on the present, is very different from the usual psychiatric focus on the past. Patients are much less concerned about understanding the origins of their complaints than about getting relief in the present and having something positive to anticipate. Mrs. K. is not interested in exploring why she is so dependent on her mother. Mrs. K. needs to feel that she can manage her life and handle her child care responsibilities.

There have been several influential advocates for practitioners engaging patients in psychotherapeutic relationships.[29,31] Most notable is Michael Balint, who taught practitioners to look at themselves and their interactions with patients to determine the therapeutic or countertherapeutic effects based on a psychoanalytical orientation. His seminal volume is *The Doctor, His Patient and the Illness.*[29] This text has helped many practitioners to understand important dynamics in the therapeutic encounter that interfere with or promote the patient's response to treatment. In this text and the subsequent volume, *Six Minutes for the Patient,*[39] which promotes making one really insightful comment in each medical interview, the importance of understanding the psychodynamics of both the patient's and the practitioner's personality structures is underscored from an analytical orientation. Balint[29] suggests that in order for practitioners to deal effectively with patients' psychological problems, a change in their personality may be required. We are far less ambitious! We suggest that practitioners only need to engage in specific behaviors, since changing behavior (to include cognitive processes) is much more feasible than changing personality structures.

In *The Twenty Minute Hour,*[40] Castelnuevo-Tedesco suggests that brief therapy needs to be planned in order to deal systematically with the interpersonal aspects of the patient's life. This implies a comprehensive and accurate analysis of the dynamics involved. Unfortunately, studies have not borne out the efficacy of this treatment approach by general practitioners.[41] Many practitioners may mistakenly cite the failure of this type of therapy in general medical practice as a justification for not engaging their patients psychotherapeutically. Our approach does not require *detailed* knowledge of a wide range of emotional disorders. It does not require an understanding of the etiology of the patient's discomfort. It does require the ability to recognize the symptoms and to provide psychological support for the patient's healthy functioning mechanisms.

Our approach integrates several newer techniques coming from crisis intervention, stress management, cognitive, behavioral, and existential literature. Abreaction and insight have unfortunately not been shown to be more effective in combating psychological distress than have the direct approaches we are promoting.[42]

Focus on the Patient's Strength

The essence of supportive therapeutic interventions is to restore patients' faith in their own capacity to take charge of their lives in a productive and satisfying way. Every difficult situation is a variation on some previous situation. If patients had not survived these earlier traumas, they would not be presenting themselves at this time. It is the practitioner's job to remind patients about having overcome past obstacles. This enhances the sense of coherence.[43] Then together they can factor out those techniques previously found successful. If patterns have consistently been destructive, then patients must be encouraged to make small changes in the ways that they would normally react in order to achieve more positive outcomes.

Each of us has a rather limited behavioral repertoire. In any situation, there is some way that we naturally respond because that is what we have learned to do under those circumstances. We tell ourselves the story that this will work. When we do not get the expected or desired result, we often redouble our efforts and keep doing whatever we are doing, longer and harder, becoming more and more frustrated when we continue to fail to achieve our ends. We have what psychologists call a limited *response set*. The practitioner can suggest that the patient make a small change in the current behavioral pattern with the expectation that this might change the outcome. The resulting change can be expected to be positive. Again, where the psychiatrist might focus on exploring why and how these behavioral patterns developed, we prefer to focus on what the patient gains when maintaining the pattern in the present. If this turns out to be nothing or pain, then we encourage the patient to change the behavioral repertoire. We specifically encourage the patient to act in some new and different ways, to develop a broader response set, and to monitor the result.

Involve the Patient's Family

The primary care practitioner, having a special relationship with the patient and the patient's family, is free to invite other family members to work with the patient in addressing whatever problem is most disturbing. Where the analyst is invested in helping the patient understand reactions to significant others, we focus on making their communication more open and direct, helping patients express feelings and ask for what they want.

We provide the knowledge that patients will not always get what they want but that by identifying their desires and stating them, the probability of getting gratification is enhanced. We encourage patients to explore options with their families and teach strategies for conflict resolution and problem solving. We make everyone aware that a problem that is experienced by one member of a family has an impact on all other members of the family. We charge them to discuss the matter, listening to each other, and then to report back to us.

THERAPEUTIC APPROACH

The most important aspect of the therapeutic relationship is the practitioner's show of concern. This means concern both for the patient as a person and for the patient as a member of a family. The practitioner can show concern through the use of a variety of techniques, including the provision of empathy.

A Relationship to Support Positive Change

Carl Rogers[44] pointed out that in order for constructive personality change to take place, the following conditions need to be met and continued over time:

1. Two persons need to be in a psychological relationship in which one person is specifically dedicated to helping the other. The practitioner, in this case, should experience "unconditional positive regard" for the patient.

2. The person in the therapeutic role experiences an empathetic understanding of the patient's internal frame of reference and is able to communicate this understanding along with the positive regard to the patient "at least to a minimum degree."

Practitioners need to make a personal commitment to helping patients cope with the emotional aspects of their lives. This commitment may entail editing the story of what it means to be a good practitioner. People tell us that we are redefining the job of primary care practitioner. That is probably true, and it is precisely what the public is demanding. Making the choice to engage the patient around life issues establishes the psychological relationship that Carl Rogers lists as the first prerequisite for therapeutic change. It also demonstrates the positive regard that the practitioner feels for the patient. This commitment becomes actualized by the practitioner's inquiring how the patient is feeling about what is going on in his or her life, establishing the context of the visit, and redefining the limits of the practitioner's interest. Having determined how the patient feels, and what he or she is most concerned about, the practitioner communicates understanding of the patient's affective state through making an empathetic response. Rogers' second condition has now been met.

If this process is repeated during every patient visit, the cumulative effect can be positive change in the patient's self-image and ability to cope constructively.

Exploration of Options

The second basic technique that practitioners can incorporate into a brief office visit is to ask patients about their options. In many cases people who are caught in a painful emotional situation are not aware that there are always options. Naturally, each potential choice has consequences, but awareness of the power to choose (even if it only affects our attitude) makes us feel less impotent and overwhelmed.

In the early 70s, Stanley Milgram[45] performed an experiment to determine people's response to authority. An experimenter demanded that subjects behave in a manner that appeared to put another person at great risk. The experiment was disguised as a learning task, and the subjects were ordered to apply shock to a stooge, who pretended to be adversely affected by this treatment. Subjects routinely followed orders although they showed discomfort, especially after passing into a range of shock marked "danger." A movie was made in which the interactions among subject, experimenter, and stooge could be observed. Although most subjects performed as directed when they were simply told, "You must continue with the experiment," in those cases where the experimenter added, "You have no choice," subjects invariably stopped, thought for a few moments, and then said something to the effect that of course they had a choice. They could walk out. And then they walked out. It seemed that just having the word "choice" mentioned made them aware that there were options.

Most people looking back on what seem to have been serious mistakes made during turning points in their lives will say that it never occurred to them that there were other options. There are always options if we take the time to look for them. It is extremely helpful to remind patients that they generally have choices, one of which is not to decide at that particular time; to choose not to choose, at least for the present. Having the practitioner suggest that there are options, that the patient can go home and list them and come back to discuss things further, is a powerful therapeutic technique.

Encouragement of New Behavior

Another powerful technique is to encourage patients to change certain behavioral patterns and engage in potentially more productive interactions with others. Although we discourage giving specific advice (the practitioner should not take responsibility for solving the patient's problem and give the patient the opportunity to sabotage), the practitioner can propose strategies that promote new behavior. These strategies might include exercising the option of taking time out or deciding not to decide; expressing feelings and asking directly for what is wanted; keeping a journal to document periods of heightened stress, noting relevant eating or sleeping patterns; and starting a regular exercise program. Once patients become aware of their power to change their behavior and receive subsequent reinforcement from the environment, these positive changes will be sustained. The patient's verbal commitment to the practitioner that certain new ways of acting will be adopted in specific situations will give the patient a powerful push in new and constructive directions.

Normalizing Reactions

The practitioner's acceptance of the patient's difficulties in handling a particular situation can be a great source of relief. The practitioner makes what have been called ubiquity statements. These pronouncements point out that people who are undergoing situations similar to what the patient is experiencing will react by feeling overwhelmed and acting in potentially destructive ways. This is called "normalizing the patient's reaction." Stating that under these circumstances anybody would feel very angry or that it is reasonable to want to walk out and let the other people cope with the mess makes the patient feel more competent. When patients understand that under certain circumstances (e.g., unemployment, bereavement, birth of a child, accidents, separation, divorce, illness, promotion, moving, graduating, child launching) people are naturally more vulnerable and easily go on *tilt*, they start to feel more comfortable with their own reactions. Once they recognize that their responses are within normal limits, it will be much easier for them to control their behavior. Sometimes it may be necessary to explain to patients that their children, spouses, or employers also have needs and that it may be necessary for the patient to come to terms with undesired changes in their interpersonal environment. It is important to reassure patients that it is not necessary to like these situations. It is only necessary to make adjustments and to deal with them. Conversely, patients need to learn that sometimes they can have strong emotional reactions to people or events without having to *do anything* about them. This can be very freeing.

Anticipatory Guidance

One of the most promising therapeutic opportunities available to the primary care practitioner is the ability to give anticipatory guidance. Anticipating problems allows people to devise strategies to cope with these problems before they arise. It also gives them time to readjust their attitudes if necessary. When situations are expected rather than presenting as a shock, coping will be more appropriate, meaning on a more mature level. Instead of responding by saying, "Isn't this awful," the patient will realize, "Goodness, I feel just like the doctor said I might. Isn't that interesting?!"

Since the practitioner sees the patient over time, anticipatory guidance about normal life cycle crises or other situations can be incorporated into routine visits for school physicals: "Have you thought about how you're going to feel when Mary is in school all day?" "How do you suppose you're going to feel once Sam, Jr., goes off to college?" During prenatal visits the practitioner can remark, "You know, having a baby is going to change many aspects of your life. You and Henry need to carefully plan in order to ensure private time for the two of you." During general physicals the practitioner can comment, "This promotion is going to involve a lot of travel, as I hear it. Have you discussed with Debbie how this will affect your relationship?" "Now that you are going back to school, I would encourage you to plan to spend quality time with each of the children regularly. You do not need to feel guilty about spending less time, if you make sure that they each get some direct positive attention daily." "Jane, now that you are going to be alone, you may find it very difficult at first. You may have trouble sleeping and not have much appetite. I expect that there will be times that you will be overcome by angry feelings for Charles. That is all perfectly normal, although right this instant that doesn't make you feel any better."

Intervening Early in the Process

Probably the most significant difference in approach between the primary care practitioner and the psychiatrist is that the practitioner sees the patient much earlier in the process of a developing problem, usually for medical symptoms. This can make a significant difference. In the case of recurrent depressions, for example, early interventions with a combination of pharmacotherapy and psychotherapy have been shown to shorten the overall length of the depressive episode by four to five months.[46] Early intervention in acute stress disorder has been shown to prevent posttraumatic stress disorder.[47] Although medication for panic attacks and other anxiety disorders is available, early application of behavioral and cognitive therapy is often recommended.[48] Identifying problems in an early stage has other advantages. Attempts that we make to solve a problem often become more of a problem than the original difficulty.[49] Drinking to forget our troubles or to relieve anxiety, running away, making threats that are taken seriously, holding feelings in, setting unenforceable limits, and engaging in power struggles are only a few examples. The practitioner's intervention at a time when the situation is still fluid can often prevent dire consequences (primary prevention), reduce the severity of consequences (secondary prevention), or at least prevent further complications (tertiary prevention).

THE BENEFIT OF BRIEF SESSIONS

The most obvious difference between our type of therapy and the usual 50-minute therapeutic hour is the time limitation that we have imposed. Yes, it is beneficial to hold encounters with the patient to a quarter of an hour. When only a few minutes are spent during the regular medical interview focusing on the psychological aspects of the patient's situation, only one or two points can be made. Our experience has been that this has a very powerful positive effect. Since persons under stress have a limited capacity to concentrate and process new information, dealing with only one or two issues has the beneficial effect of preventing information overload. It also tends to make the problem seem less complex.

Setting Priorities

When patients become familiar with the practitioner's therapeutic style and expect the inquiry, another benefit is achieved. Patients learn to arrange issues in order of priority. This process of organization is helpful and therapeutic for them. It forces them to evaluate problems in terms of severity and urgency, choosing the particular issues to be brought up at each session. In looking forward to reporting about their experiences since the previous visit (while considering the limits of time), patients are forced to summarize and focus on the high points. We recommend that practitioners remember to inquire about successes as well as failures and disappointments.

Homework Is Essential

Homework is a fundamental part of the 15-minute counseling session since the brief time available must be used efficiently. By giving the patient specific assignments, the practitioner encourages self-help and new behavior, enhancing the patient's self-esteem and sense of competence. For example, patients can be asked to list options, resources, advantages, disadvantages, disagreements with significant others, things that are bothersome, previous accomplishments, or goals to be achieved. Patients can also be asked to keep journals documenting periods of being upset, diets, sleep patterns, examples of successful coping, examples of unsuccessful coping, the best thing that happened each day, the worst thing that happened each day, ongoing problems, and potential solutions for these problems. Patients can be asked to do one new thing each day.

Making contracts with patients that certify their agreement to carry out the assigned tasks enhances the effectiveness of homework assignments. The joint expectation that the patient will return with the assignment successfully completed maintains the therapeutic connection to the practitioner between visits. Assignments need to be simple and feasible. If the patient returns without having completed an assigned task, after a brief inquiry as to what obstacle arose, a new contract is made with the expectation that the patient will follow through this time. The practitioner's interest and concern are clearly demonstrated, as is the practitioner's faith in the patient's determination to tackle the assignment. By handling situations in this manner, the practitioner supports the two essential needs of the patient: the sense of personal competence and the feeling of being connected to another human being.

Promoting Independence

Brief sessions are also beneficial because they maximize patients' own resources and minimize patients' dependence on the practitioner while providing a source of support. When patients have a partner in their search for a resolution to their problems, their confidence is enhanced, especially when this partner is someone who cares enough to follow and encourage their progress. The sense of confidence and connection is beneficial for managing stress. As stated previously, however, the problem always remains the patient's. On resolution, the patient can take personal pride in his or her ability to successfully adapt to situations that might otherwise result in more deleterious consequences.

MAKING REFERRALS

Once patients become aware of some of their interpersonal or intrapersonal difficulties in certain situations, they often feel that they would like to explore their psychological functioning to a greater depth. Perhaps the behavior of one family member makes the family aware that the dynamics that have become established are not constructive and that family therapy (restructuring) is indicated. Perhaps the practitioner feels that a particular patient would benefit from seeing a counselor for lengthier sessions to work through some deep-seated conflicts. Sometimes an unresolved grief reaction needs an in-depth exploration of the elements of a complex relationship. In all these cases, the practitioner has the option of referring the patient after first reassuring the patient that he or she will continue to provide ongoing medical care and will also continue to follow and be concerned about what is happening to the patient.

Consultations with collaborating psychiatrists or other mental health providers can be extremely helpful for the practitioner both in treating patients and in determining the need for referral. In one study of patients whose somatization disorders were being managed by primary care practitioners, one psychiatric consultation reduced the quarterly health care costs of the treatment group by over 53%.[50] However, Rosenthal and his colleagues[22] confirm our experience that the most appropriate and fruitful referrals are made by those practitioners who regularly incorporate counseling into their practice. In their study, whether patients attended more than one therapy session was related to the number of visits to the primary care practitioner before the referral. In other words, if the patient had a solid relationship with the referring doctor, the patient was more likely to overcome the obstacles and stress related to entering psychotherapy.

We interpret these findings as confirming the importance of trust and continuity in the therapeutic encounter. When making referrals, the practitioner must adequately prepare the patient for the treatment, naturally choose a practitioner known to be competent and sincere, and express positive expectations to the patient regarding the outcome of therapy. Then, if the practitioner and therapist establish ongoing communication and collaborate in the patient's care, the prognosis is excellent.

SUMMARY

The practitioner's commitment to the patient is always to provide care within the scope of the practitioner's expertise. Making the type of therapeutic interventions we have outlined is well within most practitioners' expertise and can be expected to yield positive results. By refraining from analyzing or explaining the origin of behavior, and helping the patient focus on managing reactions to situations, the practitioner's approach, although highly effective, is quite different from that of a traditional psychiatrist or other mental health professional.

Differences between the therapeutic approaches of the primary care practitioner and the psychiatrist are in the areas of patient expectations and reactions; the nature of the therapeutic relationship; and the practitioner's investment in the patient's problem. Defining themselves as mental patients carries costs that patients do not incur when treated by their practitioner. Symptoms can be treated without psychiatric labels. Small doses of therapy at a time may prove quite effective. The patient does not feel rejected, and the body and mind are not separated.

The relationship with the primary care practitioner has continuity, rapport is established nonjudgmentally, and knowledge of the family enhances the practitioner's effectiveness. The practitioner's support and interest are seen as a bonus. In contrast to the psychiatrist, the primary care practitioner tries to help the patient make a reasonably comfortable adaptation to an existing situation or environment, without getting into specific technicalities of the patient's personality structure, defense mechanisms, or even family dynamics, since these are difficult to change.

The practitioner contracts to help the patient identify specific problems and expects the patient to find some constructive resolution. This conveys a positive message. The focus is almost exclusively on situations in the present and on the patient's strengths, and the focus may involve the family. The therapeutic approach consists of using empathy, exploring options, encouraging new behavior, providing explanations, and giving anticipatory guidance. Probably the most significant difference between the approach of the primary care practitioner and that of the psychiatrist is that the practitioner sees the patient much earlier in the process of a developing problem, usually for medical symptoms. This provides the primary care practitioner a unique opportunity for early intervention.

The time limit of the sessions helps the patient to set priorities, necessitates homework, and minimizes the patient's dependence on the practitioner. Referral always remains an option. It may be requested by the patient and can be facilitated by careful preparation. Collaborative care with a mental health specialist is encouraged.

REFERENCES

1. Lorenz, A.D., Mauksch, L.B., & Gawinski, B.A. Models of collaboration. *Primary Care,* 1999, *26,* 401–410.
2. Jenkins, G.C. Collaborative care in the United Kingdom. *Primary Care,* 1999, *26,* 411–422.
3. Brown, C., & Shulberg, H.C. The efficacy of psychosocial treatments in primary care: A review of randomized clinical trials. *General Hospital Psychiatry,* 1995, *17,* 414–424.

4. Hemmings, A. A systematic review of the effectiveness of brief psychological therapies in primary health care. *Families, Systems and Health*, 2000, *18*, 279–313.

5. McHugh, P.R., & Slavney, P.R. *The Perspectives of Psychiatry*. Baltimore: Johns Hopkins University Press, 1983.

6. American Psychiatric Association. *Diagnostic and Statistical Manual of Mental Disorders*, 4th ed., text revision. Washington, D.C.: American Psychiatric Association, 2000.

7. Goldberg, D.P., & Bridges, K. Somatic presentations of psychiatric illness in primary care setting. *Journal of Psychosomatic Research*, 1988, *32*, 137–144.

8. Ben-Noun, L. Characterization of patients refusing professional psychiatric treatment in a primary care clinic. *Israeli Journal of Psychiatry Related Science*, 1996, *33*(3), 167–174.

9. Behavioral Health Industries, Inc. Study reported in *APA Monitor*, July 1989, p. 30.

10. Carpenter, P.J., Morrow, G.R., Del Gaudio, A.C., & Ritzler, B.A. Who keeps the first outpatient appointment? *American Journal of Psychiatry*, 1981, *138*, 102–105.

11. Rosenberg, C., & Rayes, A. *Keeping Patients in Psychiatric Treatment*. Cambridge, Mass.: Ballinger Publishing Co., 1976.

12. Dobscha, S.K., Delucchi, K., & Yound, M.L. Adherence with referrals for outpatient follow-up from a VA psychiatric emergency room. *Community Mental Health Journal*, 1999, *35*(5), 451–458.

13. Olfson, M. Primary care patients who refuse specialized mental health services. *Archives of Internal Medicine*, 1991, *151*, 129–132.

14. Baekland, I., & Lundwall, L. Dropping out of treatment: A critical review. *Psychological Bulletin*, 1975, *82*, 738–783.

15. Morgan, D.G. "Please see and advise": A qualitative study of patients' experiences of psychiatric outpatient care. *Social Psychiatry & Psychiatric Epidemiology*, 1999, *34*(8), 442–450.

16. Koss, M.P. Length of psychotherapy for clients seen in private practice. *Journal of Consulting Clinical Psychology*, 1979, *47*, 210–212.

17. Rockwell, K.W.J., & Pinkerton, R.S. Single-session psychotherapy. *American Journal of Psychotherapy*, 1982, *36*, 32–40.

18. Bowden, C.L., Schoenfeld, L.S., & Adams, R.L. A correlation between dropout status and improvement in a psychiatric clinic. *Hospital & Community Psychiatry*, 1980, *31*, 192–195.

19. Szasz, T.S. The myth of mental illness. *American Psychologist*, 1960, *15*, 113–118.

20. Halleck, S.L. *The Politics of Therapy*. New York: Science House, 1971.

21. Gorenstein, E.E. Debating mental illness: Implications for science, medicine, and social policy. *American Psychologist*, 1984, *39*, 40–49.

22. Rosenthal, T.C., Shiffner, J.M., Lucas, C., & DeMaggio, M. Factors involved in successful psychotherapy referral in rural primary care. *Family Medicine*, 1991, *23*, 527–530.

23. Fisher, L., & Ransom, D.C. Developing a strategy for managing behavioral health care within the context of primary care. *Archives of Family Medicine*, 1997, *6*, 324–333.

24. Larson, D.L., Nguyen, T.D., Green, R.S., & Attkisson, C.C. Enhancing the utilization of outpatient mental health services. *Community Mental Health Journal*, 1983, *19*, 305–320.

25. Angyal, A. *Neurosis and Treatment: A Holistic Theory*. New York: John Wiley & Sons, 1965.

26. Bandler, R., & Grinder, J. *The Structure of Magic. I. A Book About Language and Therapy*. Palo Alto, Calif.: Science and Behavior Books, 1975.

27. Bateson, G. *Steps to an Ecology of Mind*. New York: Ballantine Books, 1972.

28. Lennard-Jones, J.E. Functional gastrointestinal disorders. *New England Journal of Medicine*, 1983, *308*, 431–435.

29. Balint, M. *The Doctor, His Patient and the Illness*. New York: International Universities Press, 1957.

30. Adler, G. The physician and the hypochondriacal patient. *New England Journal of Medicine*, 1981, *304*, 1394–1396.

31. Harrington, J.A. Some principles of psychotherapy in general practice. *Lancet*, 1957, *1*, 799–801.

32. Kaplan, S.H., Greenfield, S., & Ware, J.E., Jr. Assessing the effects of practitioner-patient interactions on the outcomes of chronic disease. *Medical Care*, 1989, *27*, S110–S127.

33. Levinson, W., Roter, D.L., Mullooly, J.P., Dull, V.T., & Frankel, R.M. The relationship with malpractice claims among primary care physicians and surgeons. *Journal of the American Medical Association*, 1997, *277*(7), 553–559.

34. Wells, K.B., Sherbourne, C.D., Schoenbaum, M., Duan, N., Meredith, L.S., Unutzer, J., Miranda, J., Carney, M., & Rubenstein, L.V. Impact of disseminating quality improvement programs for depression in managed

primary care: A randomized controlled trial. *Journal of the American Medical Association*, 2000, *283*(2), 212–220.

35. Adams, R.J., Smith, B.J., & Ruffin, R.E. Impact of the physician's participatory style in asthma outcomes and patient satisfaction. *Annals of Allergy Asthma Immunology*, 2001, *86*(3), 263–271.

36. Gaylin, W. *Caring*. New York: Alfred A. Knopf, 1976.

37. Gaylin, p. 152.

38. Nemiah, J.C. *Foundations of Psychopathology*. New York: Oxford University Press, 1961, p. 289.

39. Balint, E., & Norell, J.S. (eds.) *Six Minutes for the Patient: Interactions in General Practice Consultation*. London: Tavistock, 1973.

40. Castelnuevo-Tedesco, P. *The Twenty Minute Hour*. Boston: Little, Brown & Co., 1965.

41. Brodaty, H., & Andrews, G. Brief psychotherapy in family practice: A controlled prospective intervention trial. *British Journal of Psychiatry*, 1983, *143*, 11–19.

42. Epstein, N.B., & Vlok, L.A. Research on the results of psychotherapy: A summary of evidence. *American Journal of Psychiatry*, 1981, *138*, 1027–1035.

43. Antonovsky, A. *Health, Stress, and Coping*. San Francisco: Jossey-Bass, 1979.

44. Rogers, C.R. The necessary and sufficient conditions of therapeutic personality change. *Journal of Consulting Psychology*, 1957, *21*, 95–103.

45. Milgram, S. Behavioral study of obedience. *Journal of Abnormal and Social Psychology*, 1963, *67*, 371–378.

46. Kupfer, D.J., Frank, E., & Perel, J.M. The advantage of early treatment intervention in recurrent depression. *Archives of General Psychiatry*, 1989, *46*, 771–775.

47. Bryant, R.A., Sackville, T., Dang, S.T., Moulds, M., & Guthrie, R. Treating acute stress disorder: An evaluation of cognitive behavior therapy and supportive counseling techniques. *American Journal of Psychiatry*, 1999, *156*(11), 1780–1786.

48. Goisman, R.M., Warshaw, M.G., & Keller, M.B. Psychosocial treatment prescriptions for generalized anxiety disorder, panic disorder, and social phobia, 1991–1996. *American Journal of Psychiatry*, 1999, *156*(11), 1819–1821.

49. Watzlawick, P., Weakland, J., & Fisch, R. *Change: Principles of Problem Formation and Problem Resolution*. New York: W.W. Norton & Co., 1974.

50. Smith, G.R., Jr., Monson, R.A., & Ray, D.C. Psychiatric consultation in somatization disorder: A randomized controlled study. *New England Journal of Medicine*, 1986, *314*, 1407–1413.

CHAPTER 6

Structuring the Therapeutic Intervention

$\mathbf{A}$re we really suggesting that the patient's psychological needs should be addressed during *every* patient visit? Yes, we are! Just as there are recognized advantages to periodic health screening from an organic perspective, many benefits accrue from assessing a patient's emotional status as part of each visit. Moreover, with our technique, the patient's psychological needs can be addressed in an efficient and effective manner.

Imagine a reasonably sensitive and specific screening test that takes about one minute, uses no supplies, is noninvasive, has no harmful side effects, and is generally acceptable to patients. Imagine further that this test may pick up potentially serious problems in an early, treatable stage and can be expected to yield *at least* 30% positive results.[1,2] Finally, imagine that use of the test might provide beneficial results for the patient, that completing the test might actually be therapeutic. Would you use such a test regularly? We think so.

Of course, you would also like to charge for the test. That seems appropriate. Generally you can, since exploration of the psychosocial aspects of the patient's problems constitutes an additional level of complexity in the treatment delivered and should be coded accordingly.

DEFINING THE STRUCTURE OF THERAPY

Practitioners have a unique opportunity to address the emotional needs of their patients, but regardless of their importance, these needs must be handled in a time-effective manner. The therapeutic intervention addressing the psychosocial aspect of patients' problems must be contained within the regular 15-minute medical visit. The therapeutic goal is to help patients reorganize some small aspect of their self-concept or behavior in a more comfortable, productive, or, at minimum, less destructive manner. The healing grows out of the established practitioner-patient relationship.

The specific treatment attempts to modify patients' images of themselves, their problems, and their options by adjusting their *assumptive world view,* the story they tell themselves about the way things are. Good interviewing techniques, a caring manner, and genuine interest demonstrated by paying serious attention and concentrating on the patient's problems pave the way toward establishing a therapeutic milieu. In the process, patients feel supported and less stressed and are able to raise their level of self-esteem as well as reengage their healthier coping styles.[3] Not only does the practitioner gain a healthier and more reasonable patient, but also this technique, with its small investment of time during each patient visit, may save the practitioner a tremendous amount of time in some future encounter. If a patient's psychological needs are not addressed and are compounded over time, they can present as monumental problems that will overextend the practitioner's resources at a subsequent visit.

DETERMINING THE CONTEXT OF THE VISIT

Optimally, every physical complaint or office visit should be seen in the context of the patient's and his or her family's total life situation. This means that in addition to descriptions of presenting symptoms, which may well represent a response to situational stress, the practitioner must determine what is going on in the patient's life as part of the history of the present illness.

Nowadays, most primary care practitioners organize their charts around the problem-oriented medical record.[4] Problems are listed and notes are arranged in *SOAP* fashion. Most practitioners are familiar with this system, which classifies progress notes into subjective, objective, assessment, and plan elements.

In order to understand patients' problems in the context of their total life situation, primary care practitioners need a larger concept of *SOAP*.[5] The total package of patient assessment requires determination of the background situation, the patient's affect, what is troubling the patient, and how the patient is handling the stress, and assessment is followed by an empathic response.[6]

BATHE

The acronym "BATHE" connotes memory jogs for the protocol to determine the context of the visit. It can also be viewed as an informal screening test for emotional problems.

B stands for background. A simple question, "What is going on in your life?" will elicit the context of the patient's visit.

A stands for affect (the feeling state). "How do you feel about that?" "How does that make you feel?" or "What's your mood?" allows the patient to report the current feeling state.

T stands for trouble. "What about the situation troubles you the most?" helps both the practitioner and the patient focus on the subjective meaning of the situation.

H stands for handling. "How are you handling that?" gives an assessment of functioning.

E stands for empathy. A response such as "That must be very difficult for you" legitimizes the patient's reaction.

Following the gathering of information, the empathetic response reassures the patient that the practitioner has understood the situation and accepts the patient's response as reasonable, given the circumstances. This is all that is minimally required to make the patient feel supported. At the same time, the technique will also enable the practitioner to identify depression, anxiety, or other disturbing symptoms. It is useful to discuss each of the elements of BATHE separately.

"B" Is for Background

The opening question of the BATHE sequence addresses what has been happening in the patient's life. If the patient complains about a problem that started perhaps two weeks previously, then the question becomes "What was going on in your life about that time?" We do not recommend asking if there was anything "new" or particularly stressful. Yes or no questions do not supply many bits of information, and there may or may not have been a major stress. Even with a positive response, we always caution practitioners not to encourage patients to tell them more about the situation, because that will use up precious time, without leading to any useful outcome. Although it is useful to determine what might have precipitated the patient's problem, the background question is probably the least important of the BATHE questions. Often patients will deny any particular stress. They may say that nothing has been going on—or perhaps just the "same old thing." Regardless of the patient's answer to the first question, it is most effective to go directly to question 2: "How does that make you feel?"

"A" Is for Affect

Asking patients how they feel about what is going on in their lives serves several important functions. In the first place it satisfies one of the critical requirements of the patient-centered interview,[7] addressing the patient's emotional response. Often patients are not in touch with their emotional response. Illness behavior is a universal mechanism used by people with psychological disturbance to express their distress and seek medical care.[8-10] Helping patients get in touch with and express their feelings directly is highly therapeutic. Once expressed, feelings do not have to be "somatized." When patients are labeling their feelings, they should be encouraged to use adjectives such as mad, glad, sad, disappointed, frustrated, devastated, or guilty. Sometimes patients will use the phrase "I feel" to express a judgment. Anytime you can substitute the phrase "I think" for the words "I feel," that is not a feeling. Feelings are whatever feelings are. They are neither good nor bad, but that individual's response to the particular situation. Feelings need not be justified or explained; they just have to be accepted. Many people are uncomfortable with the feelings they have. It is highly therapeutic to give people permission to feel the way they feel. In the BATHE sequence, the practitioner uses attentive listening and body language to make the patient feel accepted. If the patient is having a problem labeling a feeling, the practitioner may wish to suggest that under similar circumstances many people would feel angry, frustrated, overwhelmed, or whatever an appropriate response might be.

"T" Is for Trouble

This is the most important of the BATHE questions. "What about the situation troubles you the most?" helps the patient to get in touch with the meaning of the situation. This question generally requires the patient to stop and think. Many people are not particularly self-reflecting without some coaching. It has been our experience that confronted with the question "What about that troubles you?" patients often have an "Aha!" reaction and realize something that had been out of their awareness until that time. Practitioners are often surprised by the answers that this question elicits, since people have highly unique reactions to common situational circumstances. Because what is most troubling about the situation constitutes definition of the problem, arriving at some constructive solution now becomes possible. When patients relate some positive event in their lives and a positive feeling to accompany it, it is still useful to ask whether anything about the situation troubles the patient, since ambivalence is a common experience. This allows the patient to express reservations that may or may not be significant but need to be addressed.

"H" Is for Handling

This question can be used in different ways. Asking "How are you handling that?" gives the practitioner valuable information about possibly destructive behaviors that the patient may be using to cope. Often the patient will reply, "not very well" and list some of the symptoms that prompted the office visit and then wonder if perhaps the situation precipitated those reactions. In other words, the (Socratic) questioning allows patients to get in touch with answers they already have but are not aware of.

Sometimes it is more efficacious to ask, "How could you handle that?" This intervention empowers patients to arrive at solutions they may not have considered previously. The implication is that they are capable of dealing with the situation constructively. Later chapters will discuss a variety of tasks that can be assigned as homework to help patients come to positive resolution of their problems.

"E" Is for Empathy

It is crucial that practitioners finish the BATHE sequence with a statement that demonstrates understanding and empathy. Acknowledging the difficulty of the situation, the fact that the patient is doing the best that can be expected under the circumstances or that this is obviously very painful, validates the patient's experience and makes him or her feel competent and connected in a positive way to the practitioner. It provides effective psychological support. It also closes the inquiry and allows the practitioner to move back to the physical aspects of the patient's problem.

In a majority of cases, when the BATHE technique is used, situational factors are identified, feelings are validated, meaning is assessed, a plan is made, and psychological support is provided. Nothing further is required. The intervention is complete. The whole interaction usually takes less than one minute.

When Is It Best to BATHE?

When practitioners apply the BATHE technique early in the interview, an effective and efficient psychotherapeutic intervention is structured into every patient encounter. The context of the visit has been incorporated into the session, patients' emotional reactions are addressed, and there is closure. A basic screening for anxiety or depressive disorders has also been accomplished. Sometimes there may not be a problem, but having the opportunity for social intercourse is still gratifying for the patient.[11,12] Most of the time, patients reveal some ongoing concern. Often the patient feels better immediately after completion of the BATHE protocol, having become aware of the underlying issue that makes a situation problematic. The practitioner's interest and empathic response make the patient feel connected. Sorting out the problem and the notion of "handling it" makes the patient feel more competent. The practitioner then proceeds with further medical history and the appropriate physical examination. When the routine BATHE interaction uncovers a serious problem, additional support and/or provision for follow-up or referral is structured into the latter part of the visit, as shown by the following example:

A 34-year-old woman, who had been a patient at the family practice center for about one year, presented in the office complaining about a vaginal discharge. She appeared to be quite agitated. Dr. W., who was a second-year resident at the time, inquired about what was going on in her life. The patient started to cry.

"I just found out that my husband has been having an affair with my oldest sister for the past year and a half."

"How do you feel about that?" (The physician felt a little foolish. It seemed like this was an inane question to ask under the circumstances, but he really did not know what else to ask.)

"I feel angry. I have mood swings. I go up and down. I also feel depressed."

After taking several deep breaths to center himself, Dr. W. asked what about the situation troubled the patient the most. She replied, "I have two children. They are two and five, and I really don't want to be a single parent."

(The physician was surprised. He would have expected her to be most troubled because of the familial involvement, the betrayal, or the time frame.)

"How are you handling it?" was his final question.

The patient stated that she was handling things very badly. She was angry and did a lot of shouting at her husband. She also added that she was afraid that the children were starting to be affected, she was very short-tempered with them, and they really did not deserve that.

The physician was taken aback by this history. Still, he managed to respond, "That sounds like a horrendous situation."

"Yes, it is," said the patient and visibly relaxed.

"Why don't we examine you now and find out what we can do about your vaginal discomfort," said the physician, "and then we'll talk some more."

Patients' Understanding of Stress

Happily not all situations are as dramatic or traumatic as the above example. In our practice BATHE is used routinely and uncovers a variety of situations, more often chronic than acute. Our experience has been that the technique is well accepted by patients, even those coming from a variety of cultures. Once confronted by a focused question, patients are often acutely aware of the role of stress in precipitating their symptoms. Consider the following description of a visit reported by a psychology intern who had monitored the encounter over closed-circuit television:

Ms. K. is a middle-aged African-American female, a Rutgers student, who has come to the office for an initial visit. Her presenting problem is a dry scalp with associated peeling and flaking. She reports that she has been experiencing this problem for several weeks but that lately it seems to have worsened. She appears pleasant and cooperative during the discussion of her symptomatology and throughout the subsequent physical examination by the physician. However, she offered no complaints regarding situational stressors or issues of concern in her life.

When the doctor specifically *asked what was going on in the patient's life*, she responded by saying she was an older woman and was currently back in school. The physician then *asked how she felt about this*. The patient seemed slightly uncomfortable disclosing her feelings and focused instead on discussing the content of her college program. The physician listened intently for a brief while. Then he patiently *asked again how she felt about that*. Ms. K.'s shoulders appeared to relax as she admitted to feeling rather stressed out concerning the challenges of returning to school later in life. The physician then commented that *that must be very difficult for her*. The patient nodded her head in agreement and seemed relieved to have her feelings validated.

The doctor then asked *what troubled the patient the most about her situation*. The patient disclosed that she found the workload and associated stress and anxiety most disconcerting. The doctor then *inquired how the patient had been handling the anxiety*. The patient shared laughter with the doctor as she replied that a lot of prayers had been getting her through.

The physician acknowledged the helpfulness of prayer and then also introduced the importance of exercise as a further means of reducing her stress. Ms. K. reported that she used to exercise but had not lately. The doctor then explained, "The reason that I am asking about your stress is that there is a mind-body connection and often psychological issues can manifest as or exacerbate physical problems such as with your scalp." This appeared to strike a responsive chord with the patient as she related, "Oh, yes, Doctor, in fact a few years ago when I was going through a stressful divorce, I remember having similar problems with my scalp." The discussion then returned to the topic of exercise, and with the patient's eager collaboration, together they formulated a daily exercise regimen that could realistically be implemented given the rigorous demands of Ms. K.'s scholastic program.

In this situation, the physician wove BATHE into the encounter and was able to use it to help the patient make sense of her symptoms as well as prescribing and getting agreement for an effective management plan.

SUPPORTING THE PATIENT

In Chapter 2 we defined social support as a psychological mechanism that provides positive information to the individual about his or her interaction with other people. More technically in social science studies social support has been defined as "the sum of the social, emotional and instrumental exchanges with which the individual is involved having the subjective consequence that an individual sees him or herself as an object of continuing value in the eyes of significant others."[13] Certainly, the interaction between the patient and the practitioner involves social, emotional, and instrumental exchanges. It is obviously important that practitioners behave in such a manner that patients get the impression that they are seen as individuals who have continuing value in the eyes of the practitioner. Social support has been shown to be critical in mitigating the effects of various stressors.[14] Social support is demonstrated by engaging in one or more of the following behaviors: (1) an expression of positive affect, (2) an endorsement of the person's behavior, perception, or expressed views, (3) giving symbolic or material aid, and (4) giving the opportunity to express feelings in an accepting atmosphere.

It is clear that when practitioners incorporate BATHE into every patient visit, many of the above criteria will be satisfied. Interest and positive affect have been expressed, and feelings have been accepted. Information is gathered that helps both patient and practitioner understand the situation and the patient's reaction to it, and the diagnosis becomes a large part of the cure. Clearly defining the problem helps focus the patient and the practitioner on the resources necessary to reach an acceptable resolution.

Dealing With Multiple Problems

Often the practitioner encounters multiple problems in the course of interviewing a patient. Here, again, having a practical structure for dealing with these problems is helpful both in keeping the practitioner focused and in meeting the patient's needs. If an unexpected emotional response occurs during the interview, the practitioner finds out what is going on, explores the issue with three questions, and effects closure with an empathic statement. In this way, a simple technique, sequentially applied, can effectively be used to handle complex situations. The following case, reported by one of our senior residents, illustrates the principles we are promoting:

A new patient, a 38-year-old woman, presented with multiple concerns, including contraception, vaginal itching, dyspareunia, and frequent headaches. On further questioning, she was a working mother of three teenage children, widowed six years previously, and remarried one year ago. Family history was positive for hypertension and diabetes in her grandparents and multiple sclerosis (MS) in her mother. The mother was currently 56 years old and had been in a nursing home for 12 years. At this point in the interview, the patient appeared tearful but attempted to suppress the tears. I asked her what was going on and then used the rest of the BATHE technique. The patient started to cry, saying that she had not cried for years about her mother. I asked her what her mom had been like. She stated she had always admired her mother's energy and unselfishness, which was why she felt so guilty about having her in the nursing home. I empathized, and we went on. Subsequently, I found out that her mother's diagnosis had been made at the age of 38. I asked her what she thought might be causing her headaches. She said I shouldn't think she was crazy, but she had considered whether it might not be MS. I supported her by telling her that that was a natural concern under the circumstances and that I would do a thorough evaluation in that regard.

At this point, about 10 minutes into the interview, I pointed out that she had come with quite a few concerns and asked her which one she wanted most to deal with in this visit. She stated that she was most concerned about her vaginal itch. After some routine questions regarding the genitourinary (GU) system, I asked how this condition was affecting her sexuality, to which she replied that she and her husband had not slept together in six months! She stated that she suspected him of having an affair. Six months ago also corresponded to the anniversary of her first husband's death. I asked a background question about the circumstances of her marriage and again finished the BATHE sequence. I then asked her to prepare for the physical examination and assured her I would check for venereal disease. She appeared relieved and revealed that she had also had a "fling" just before the onset of the itching.

During the physical exam, I did enough of a review of systems to assure myself that her headaches were not of an immediately serious nature, and I reassured her regarding her pelvic exam. I supported her by stating that she seemed to be handling things well under such stressful circumstances. I asked her to make an appointment for evaluation of her headaches and further discussion of her other concerns, including contraception. I asked her if she had any questions, and she said no but that she was very relieved after talking with me. The entire session lasted 25 minutes.

In this case, the practitioner sequentially dealt with a variety of problems, related to both present circumstances and unresolved grief from the past. By repeatedly using the BATHE structure, she dealt with these problems in a timely, effective, and sensitive manner.

The Resistant Patient

Certainly there are patients who are highly invested in separating their body symptoms from their emotional states. Somatization is commonly seen in primary care across cultures and is generally associated with significant health problems and disabilities.[8] A few patients may be taken aback when questioned by their practitioners about what is going on in their lives. They may respond with "nothing." The practitioner has several choices when this happens. First, the subject can be dropped. We do not recommend this, because it reinforces somatization and wastes an opportunity to help the patient learn to connect physical conditions to emotional states. The second option, to repeat the word "nothing" with a questioning inflection, often results in the patient hesitantly revealing some current problem or a list of chronic annoyances. The rest of the BATHE sequence is then followed. The third option is simply to continue with the BATHE protocol, asking how the patient feels about the fact that nothing is going on. Practitioners tell us that they get some fascinating responses, such as the following common examples: "Just dreadful. I'm bored to tears." "Kind of mad, I guess. I'm tired of the same old thing!" "Awful. By now I was expecting to be promoted and nothing has happened." Regardless of the patient's reaction, BATHE usually provides important insights for the patient, as the following case illustrates:

A 29-year-old woman came to the Family Practice Center complaining of having had a headache for four days. Her past history included headaches that started 12 years previously and recurred intermittently around the time of her period. After getting a complete description of her symptoms and the history of the present illness, the resident, who was not the patient's regular doctor, asked her what was going on in her life. She replied, "nothing." "How do you feel about that?" he continued as taught. "How am I supposed to feel with nothing going on?" He tried one more time. "What about it troubles you the most?" She seemed exasperated, "What is supposed to trouble me when there is nothing going on in my life?" The resident dropped the subject and proceeded with his exam.

Discussion of the case with the preceptor led to the conclusion that, in spite of the patient's denial, this was most likely a muscle tension headache, probably precipitated by stress or conflict. A decision was made to treat. When the resident went back into the examination room and gave the patient her prescription for an analgesic, he gently posited, "There is something going on in your life, isn't there? You just don't want to talk with me about it."

The patient looked at him with admiration and smiled slightly. He suggested that she might want to come back and talk with her regular doctor. The resident felt terrific. There had been a moment of real communication. He was sure that the patient had felt it also.

WHEN THE PATIENT COMES BACK TO TALK

Subsequent chapters will provide many specific suggestions and techniques for use in a 15-minute visit. At this point, let us look briefly at how Dr. Alan Buchanan, a psychiatrist at the University of British Columbia, has used the BATHE protocol to teach primary care physicians how to structure a 10-minute "counseling session."[15]

B stands for background. The opening two minutes belong to the patient. You open with "Tell me what's been going on since our last visit." The underlying message is that the practitioner is there to listen to the patient—and there is no need to rush.

A stands for affect (the feeling state). Summarize the feelings. The underlying message is "I have been listening." Dr. Buchanan suggests that since many patients cannot label feelings on their own, this can be very helpful to them.

T stands for trouble. "What is the worst thing about this situation?" The underlying message is a combination of "we can talk about anything here" and "our time is short so we must focus."

H stands for handling. "And how did you handle this?" sends the message that "you can handle this situation." What is important here is to manage this crisis, not to get stuck in overwhelming feelings.

E stands for empathy. Normalize the patient's reaction to the crisis. "It sounds awful, and I agree with what you have done so far—anybody would have had problems with this situation."

In the final few minutes, the physician asks, "What is the best thing that has happened lately?" Dr. Buchanan comments that this sometimes injects humor or initiates the process of seeing the crisis as an opportunity for change. Then the physician states, "For the next time I'd like you to (write the problem out in detail, or write down some options available, or reach out to some specific sources of support)." The underlying message is "You *can* handle this situation."

He ends the interview with a closing statement: "I'm glad we had a chance to talk about this," "I feel like I know you better," or just "Sorry, but our time is up for today."

More will be said in Chapter 8 about how to structure visits when the patient comes back to talk.

THE USE OF MEDICATION

One of the beauties of providing psychotherapeutic intervention in primary care is the option to combine talk therapy with medication. The individual practitioner must determine how and when to prescribe pharmacological treatment to ease the patient's symptoms. Chapter 9 will focus on specific treatments that can be part of the practitioner's armamentarium. In general, if patients' acute distress is so severe as to seriously interfere with their functioning, we recommend using medication to alleviate their symptoms. When patients are not able to sleep, it is difficult to restore some measure of equilibrium. In treating depression, the practitioner has the option of prescribing psychotropic medication along with providing supportive therapy. Unfortunately, studies show that doctors do not necessarily talk with patients often once a diagnosis is made and a prescription issued.[16] It is critical to help patients develop realistic expectations about the action of the medication as well as to help them to handle the problematic aspects of their current situations. Although comparative outcome studies continue to challenge researchers, according to the literature over the last 20 years, the combination of medical and psychological treatment is generally more effective than either modality by itself.[17-19]

Although medication can be extremely useful in managing acute problems, treating symptoms without addressing the underlying causes of a chronic problem perpetuates a patient's sense of powerlessness and hopelessness. A prescription for alprazolam (Xanax) does nothing to fix a bad marriage where communications have broken down. Patients need to be mobilized to change their behavior. If the patient is requesting medication, however, this provides an opportunity to bond with the patient. Later, an ongoing negotiation may be required to taper the medication over time.

DIFFERENTIATING APPROACHES FOR CHRONIC AND ACUTE PROBLEMS

The BATHE technique is useful for determining whether a problem is chronic or acute. Different approaches depend on this classification.[20] There are also different underlying stories that must be considered.

Treating Acute Conditions

The medical model lends itself quite well to dealing with acute situations and with very dependent patients. The underlying story in acute situations is that the patient is not to blame for creating the problem—the patient is sick. The practitioner therefore takes responsibility for finding a solution for the problem: to diagnose, counsel, suggest, prescribe, and give orders that must be followed. All that is required of the patient is to comply with the treatment. This helps the patient to feel secure. The more acute the problem, the more important for the practitioner to take charge, at least temporarily. The practitioner makes suggestions and guides the patient in handling the situation. Close follow-up is important so that the patient feels supported and connected. In an emergency situation, and emergency for the patient is a subjective state, authoritarian behavior relieves anxiety. Ultimately, however, responsibility and control need to be returned to the patient.

Managing Chronic Problems

When dealing with chronic problems a useful approach also employs the story that patients are not to blame for creating their problems. They may have been abused, uninformed, or otherwise deprived. Perhaps it was circumstance, karma, bad parenting, some unavoidable breakdown, inexperience, or just bad judgment. Regardless, this story says that the patient is responsible for effecting solutions. This can be accomplished by asking for and accepting help, coping constructively with the problem, and using it as a learning opportunity. In dealing with patients who are having chronic problems, this is a very useful approach. The removal of blame for creation of the problem is therapeutic. It relieves guilt and raises the patient's level of self-esteem. Although no blame is placed for developing chronically difficult situations, the patient is expected to take responsibility for dealing with these problems constructively and finding solutions. The practitioner will help, be a sounding board, and lead the cheering section, but the patient retains responsibility for managing the problem. The practitioner's positive expectation regarding the patient's ability to resolve the problem—the infusion of hope—is a powerful therapeutic tool.

Actually, the practitioner may believe the patient to be responsible for creating the problem, as in the case of the 38-year-old woman who had had a "fling"; however, pointing this out is rarely therapeutic since it underscores the patient's sense of hopelessness, guilt, and self-deprecation. Relieving patients of blame allows them to direct their energies outward, to work on solving their problems or transforming their environments without wasting energy berating themselves for creating these problems or permitting others to create them.[15]

As we have seen, determining whether a problem is chronic or acute allows the practitioner to choose the more effective therapeutic strategy. In either case, the focus is on dealing with the problem. In general, empowering patients and holding them responsible for finding solutions foster self-esteem. However, when patients are in crisis, the practitioner may want to take a more active role and satisfy dependency needs. In either case, the patient feels better and functions better. Because the focus is always on helping the patient change the outcome, either approach combats the pessimistic explanatory style characterized by the story that the situation is caused by internal, stable, and global factors and can never be fixed.[21]

Aiming for Small Wins

In previous chapters we have pointed out that it is the feeling of powerlessness, or of demoralization, that brings the patient to a therapist.[22] It is feeling helpless in the face of threat that is devastating, physically and mentally.[23,24] In many cases, the overwhelming scope of problems faced by individuals, and for that matter, by society as a whole, predisposes people to feeling helpless, since there appears to be little that can be done to effect any kind of meaningful solution. According to K.E. Weick,[25] attempted large-scale solutions to overwhelming societal problems, such as crime, traffic congestion, and pollution, often create new problems, such as the need for increased law enforcement;

removal of needed funds from other services; multilane highways drawing more people away from mass transit; and the cost of pollution control, raising taxes. The most detrimental aspect of the situation, however, is that people's level of arousal gets raised without their having access to responses that will effectively impact the situation. This is the essence of *stress*. People go on overload because they perceive the severity and intensity of the problem while feeling helpless to do anything about it.

The corrective strategy proposed by Weick[25] is to focus on minor leverage points that enable people to engage in productive problem solving. In other words, people can act to make other people aware of the problem, organize rallies, write letters, wear red, white, and blue ribbons, get attention from the newspapers, and in that way feel as though they are accomplishing something. They are not just standing idly by, watching the world go to ruin.

Achieving small wins has the effect of reversing both the overarousal and apathy that result from feeling demoralized. Focusing patients on small wins provides practical, immediate, and surprisingly effective results, since it lowers their levels of psychological distress, that is, gets them off *tilt*. This is a therapeutic milestone. Getting patients to focus on a minor change in their own behavior—slightly changing a schedule, carving out time for themselves, organizing a list, clearly asking for something they want, calling a friend, expressing feelings without attacking or blaming, writing a letter, or even sending a postcard—can result in a small win. Successfully doing one little task provides a sense of having some power, and there is less risk for patients when they tackle a problem in stages, since less is riding on each particular behavior. Not only is the outcome more likely to be positive, but also it will be less traumatic if it is not. The main idea is to make patients aware that their actions can make a difference. Weick explained as follows:

> Brief therapy is most successful when the client is persuaded to do just one thing differently that interdicts the pattern of attempted solutions up to that point. Extremely easy or extremely difficult goals are less compelling than are goals set closer to perceived capabilities. Learning tends to occur in small increments rather than in an all-or-none fashion.[26]

Small wins increase the chance of success, foster optimism, help people to refocus their energy productively, and restore belief in personal control. The effectiveness of the intervention grows out of the practitioner's faith in the patient's ability to effect small, meaningful changes.

Engaging the Patient in a Psychotherapeutic Contract

After physical examination and medical management decisions have been made, the practitioner returns to the psychosocial aspects. Determining the nature of the problem and giving an empathic response constitute a psychotherapeutic intervention. As has been stated, it focuses the patient and legitimizes his or her feelings. The practitioner now suggests that regardless of the origin of the problem, little can be gained by placing blame. Rather, it is important to determine what can be done and to evaluate the available options to manage the situation. The practitioner becomes the patient's ally in dealing with the problem. One approach is to advise the patient to take some time to think about it and return in one or two weeks if the problem is not resolved. If a patient is feeling overwhelmed and problems are numerous and complex, a contract, specifically a verbal understanding, is made for follow-up. It is helpful to specify that the practitioner will meet with the patient for a particular number of sessions.

Chapter 10 will discuss specific considerations that must be applied to patients presenting with certain problems, or perhaps we should say certain problem patients: hypochondriacal, depressed, suicidal, or grieving patients. All these lend themselves to therapeutic intervention by the primary care practitioner, provided that the contract is made clear. The practitioner's role, commitment, and limitations must be clearly spelled out. The patient's responsibilities must also be stated, acknowledged, and documented in the chart. Once a patient recognizes the need for a therapeutic process, referral to a mental health professional providing collaborative care is a superb option. Anytime the practitioner feels overwhelmed by the extent of the patient's problems, a psychiatric consult or referral is indicated. Patients to be referred include psychotic, addicted, or violent patients or any patient whose condition makes the practitioner feel uncomfortable. When referring a patient, there is an understanding that the practitioner will continue to be involved with the patient and continue to provide ongoing medical care.

Determining Number Of Sessions

We know from crisis theory, as described by Gerald Caplan,[27] that an intense crisis situation is usually resolved in six to eight weeks. As discussed in Chapter 2, crisis is a time of major stress as people try to adapt to large-scale acute or anticipated change. During a period of crisis, patients tend to function much less efficiently than they normally do. People under stress regress to more primitive modes of behavior, have a narrower view, have a harder time with problem solving, and are not able to see potential options.[25] The practitioner's expressed support engages the patient's sense of well-being and provides an ally to help with the problem. In making a contract for follow-up, the practitioner commits to following the patient through the time of greatest stress. From crisis theory, it is obvious that six or eight weeks provides a reasonable expectation of problem resolution. The practitioner arranges to see the patient regularly during that time. Once each week is appropriate if the problem is serious. Once every other week is sufficient if the patient is less overwhelmed. If the patient is feeling totally unstrung, a twice-weekly contact may be necessary during the acute phase of the crisis.

By agreeing to see the patient regularly and briefly for a specified number of sessions, the practitioner conveys the message that the problem is solvable and that the practitioner expects resolution to come within a reasonable period of time. Conveying this message is part of the therapeutic intervention. Hope is engaged, since patients recognize that the practitioner is seeing factors that mitigate their feelings of despair. Perhaps the problem is manageable after all. Patients regain a sense of worth based on the practitioner wanting to engage with them to resolve the situation. It is a consistent message. Not only is the practitioner saying that the patient is worthy and deserving, but also the practitioner is making a commitment to work with the patient. The fact that the practitioner places no blame but suggests that the problem needs to be resolved is practical.

Contracting to help the patient resolve the problem is one of the most affirming and therapeutic messages that can be conveyed. The patient has a partner and feels less isolated and less overwhelmed by the problem. Often, when the patient's morale has been restored, the problems get resolved more expeditiously than expected.

Example: The Grieving Patient

Patients are often overcome when they suffer significant losses. Traumatic grief has been shown to negatively affect both physical and psychological health.[28] When working with a bereaved patient, or discovering a situation of unresolved grief during a routine inquiry, the practitioner should explain the need for working through feelings related to significant relationships that have been terminated through death or other circumstances. Grief work can usually be accomplished in six or eight sessions.

The process of mourning requires that patients come to terms with both the positive and negative feelings related to the person who is gone. It requires the patient to reflect, remember, and process significant milestones in the relationship. Much of this work can be done by writing about the person, their history, and characteristics.[29] Patients should also be encouraged to look at photographs, talk with friends and relatives, and regularly check in with the practitioner to report on their progress. Although this can be a painful process, it is necessary in order to bring closure and allow the survivor to reengage with life.

The practitioner may contract with the patient for six or eight sessions to supervise the grief work or can refer the patient to a collaborating mental health practitioner or an ongoing support group. In any case, therapy must focus on reviewing the significant aspects of the terminated relationship, accepting the pain and finality of the loss, coming to terms with the good and bad aspects, and finally letting go.

THE EFFICACY OF TIME

Using the framework of *The Fifteen Minute Hour* the practitioner provides a special time and safe environment for the patient to tell and assess some aspect of his or her story. The patient is invited to reexamine responses to situations, look at options, chart new goals, and acquire a more positive sense of self-efficacy. The clinician helps the patient to focus on one particular problem and suggests that the patient will be able to replicate the process.

The time constraint is useful because it prevents overloading the patient and adding to the confusion. The practitioner conveys optimism that problems can be resolved one at a time and indicates that he or she is there to help the patient work through the problems. By returning to patients the sense of having some potential for affecting the course of their lives, for making their own decisions and choices, the practitioner is acting in a most highly therapeutic manner. In addition, when the practitioner routinely incorporates this approach into every patient encounter, efficiency is built into the practice. A little energy invested in this process on each visit fosters the image of the practitioner as an empathic and involved figure. As a result, the practitioner is able to handle patients' problems in an effective and timely fashion often before they assume overwhelming proportions.

ONE LAST POINT

In addition to asking patients the right questions, it is important to make sure everyone involved in the patient encounter is listening. Both the practitioner's and the patient's listening skills are vital to solving medical problems.[30]

SUMMARY

Many benefits accrue from assessing a patient's emotional status as part of each visit. Every physical complaint or office visit should be seen in the context of the patient's and his or her family's total life situation. The therapeutic effect grows out of the practitioner-patient relationship. The letters "BATHE" connote memory jobs for handling the context of the visit. "B" stands for background: "What is going on?" "A" stands for affect: "How do you feel about it?" "T" stands for trouble: "What about it bothers you most?" "H" stands for handling: "How are you dealing with that?" "E" stands for empathy: "That must be very difficult for you!"

BATHEing the patient early in the interview structures an effective and efficient psychotherapeutic intervention into every patient encounter. Multiple problems can be handled by sequentially applying the simple technique. BATHE can also be used to structure a return visit and to determine whether a problem is chronic or acute. The practitioner may wish to use medication as an adjunct to talk therapy. In acute situations it is useful for practitioners to take an active role in finding solutions, whereas chronic problems require that patients be held responsible for problem resolution. Small wins combat the patient's sense of being overwhelmed and allow patients to experience success. Incremental steps are effective in promoting change because they increase a patient's confidence.

The practitioner engages the patient in a therapeutic contract by committing to follow the psychosocial context of the patient's life. Crises can generally be resolved within six or eight weeks, which is also a good estimate for accomplishing grief work. The patient will do much of the work in writing and report the progress during regular visits. The time constraint inherent in the brief session is useful because it prevents overloading the patient. The practitioner's optimism and focus on one problem at a time are an effective strategy and provide a model for further work.

REFERENCES

1. Barsky, A.J. Hidden reasons some patients visit doctors. *Annals of Internal Medicine*, 1981, *94*, 492–498.
2. McQuaid, J.R., Stein, M.B., Laffaye, D., & McCahill, M.E. Depression in a primary care clinic: The prevalence and impact of an unrecognized disorder. *Journal of Affective Disorders*, 1999, *55*, 1–10.

3. Vaillant, G.E. *Adaptation to Life.* Boston: Little, Brown & Co., 1977.

4. Weed, L.L. *Medical Records, Medical Education, and Patient Care.* Cleveland: The Press of Case Western Reserve, 1969.

5. Kallman, H., & Stuart, M.R. BATH—A simple mnemonic to integrate psychosocial data into a soaped chart. Unpublished manuscript. 1980.

6. Tallia, A.F. Verbal communication, 1981. (Suggested adding "E for Empathy" to the acronym BATH to create the acronym BATHE.)

7. Stewart, M., Brown, J.B., Weston, W.W., McWhinney, I.R., McWilliam, C.L., & Freeman, T.R. *Patient-Centered Medicine: Transforming the Clinical Method.* Thousand Oaks, Calif.: Sage Publications, 1995.

8. Gureje, O., Simon, G.E., Ustun, T.B., & Goldberg, D.P. Somatization in cross-cultural perspective: A World Health Organization study in primary care. *American Journal of Psychiatry,* 1997, *154,* 989–995.

9. Cameron, L.D., Leventhal, H., & Leventhal, E.A. Symptom ambiguity, life stress, and decisions to seek medical care. *Psychosomatic Medicine,* 1995, *57,* 37–47.

10. Epstein, R.M., Quill, T.E., & McWhinney, I.R. Somatization reconsidered. *Archives of Internal Medicine,* 1999, *159*(3), 215–222.

11. Bertakis, K.D., Roter, D., & Putnam, S.M. The relationship of physician medical interview style to patient satisfaction. *Journal of Family Practice,* 1991, *32*(2), 175–181.

12. Roter, D. The enduring and evolving nature of the patient-physician relationship. *Patient Education and Counseling,* 2000, *39*(1), 5–15.

13. Glass, T.A., Matchar, D.B., Belyea, M., & Feussner, J.R. Impact of social support on outcome of first stroke. *Stroke,* 1993, *24*(1), 64–70.

14. House, J.S., Landis, K.R., & Umberson, D. Social relationships and health. *Science,* 1988, *241,* 540–545.

15. Buchanan, A. Counseling tips for family practitioners. In Sehon, A., & Buchanan, A. (eds.) *Syllabus from Psychiatric Update Conferences for Physicians, 1991–92.* Vancouver, B.C.: Sehon-Buchanan Medical Media, p. 82.

16. Meredith, L.S., Wells, K.B., Kaplan, S.H., & Mazel, R.M. Counseling typically provided for depression. *Archives of General Psychiatry,* 1996, *53,* 905–912.

17. Weissman, M.M. The psychological treatment of depression: Evidence for the efficacy of psychotherapy alone, in comparison with, and in combination with pharmacotherapy. *Archives of General Psychiatry,* 1979, *36,* 1261–1269.

18. Power, K.G., Simpson, R.J., Swanson, V., & Wallace, L.A. Controlled comparison of pharmacological and psychological treatment of generalized anxiety disorder in primary care. *British Journal of General Practice,* 1990, *40,* 289–294.

19. Kendall, P.C., & Lipman, A.J. Psychological and pharmacological therapy: Methods and modes for comparative outcome research. *Journal of Consulting and Clinical Psychology,* 1991, *59,* 78–87.

20. Brickman, P., Rabinowitz, V.C., Karuza, J., Jr., Coates, D., Cohn, E., & Kidder, L. Models of helping and coping. *American Psychologist,* 1982, *37,* 368–384.

21. Peterson, C., Colvin, D., & Lin, E.H. Explanatory style and helplessness. *Social Behavior and Personality,* 1992, *20,* 1–14.

22. Frank, J.D. Psychotherapy: The restoration of morale. *American Journal of Psychiatry,* 1974, *131,* 271–274.

23. Peterson, C., Seligman, M.E.P., & Vaillant, G.E. Pessimistic explanatory style as a risk factor for physical illness: A thirty-five-year longitudinal study. *Journal of Social and Personality Psychology,* 1988, *55,* 23–27.

24. Levy, S.M., Herberman, R.B., Maluish, A.M., Schlein, B., & Lippman, M. Prognostic risk assessment in primary breast cancer by behavioral and immunological parameters. *Health Psychology,* 1985, *4,* 99–113.

25. Weick, K.E. Small wins: Redefining the scale of social problems. *American Psychologist,* 1984, *39,* 40–49.

26. Weick. p. 45.

27. Caplan, G. *Principles of Preventive Psychiatry.* New York: Basic Books, 1964.

28. Prigerson, H.G., Bierhals, A.J., Kasl, S.V., Reynolds, C.F., Shear, M.K., Day, N., Beery, L.C., Newsom, J.T., & Jacobs, S. Traumatic grief as a risk factor for mental and physical morbidity. *American Journal of Psychiatry,* 1997, *154*(5), 616–623.

29. Pennebaker, J.W. Putting stress into words: Health, linguistic, and therapeutic implications. *Behavior Research and Therapy,* 1993, *31,* 539–548.

30. Lieberman, J.A., Stuart, M.R., & Robinson, S.A. Enhance the patient visit with counseling and listening skills. *Family Practice Management,* 1996, *3*(10), 70–75.

CHAPTER 7

Rationale and Techniques for 15-Minute Therapy

Patients generally assume that their practitioners are technically competent to diagnose and treat disease. Expressing interest in the patient and demonstrating warmth and support, particularly in the presence of debilitating, painful, or frightening symptoms, are an added bonus.

In one of his seminal writings McWhinney[1] pointed out that practitioners are much more adept at applying the biological and physical sciences to the practice of medicine than they are in utilizing knowledge from the behavioral sciences. Every patient with an organic illness also "exhibits some form of behavior." It is important that practitioners pay attention to this behavior, as well as to the social context of the patient's symptoms. Even when psychiatric symptoms are the chief complaint, McWhinney states that most of the emotional disorders in general medical practice fall into the category of "problems of living," that is, the natural anxiety of people who are responding to perceived threats to their health or well-being. We cannot agree more! Although a patient's response to illness is determined by many factors, including genetic makeup, early history, previous experience with illness, current life situation, and aspirations for the future, the reaction to the current life situation is probably the most amenable to alteration by the practitioner. For this reason, it is critical for the practitioner to routinely ask all patients about what is going on in their lives.

ROUTINELY INQUIRING ABOUT CURRENT LIFE SITUATIONS

Since patients' presenting problems are usually a complex amalgamation of physical, psychological, and social factors, ascertaining the situational context of the patient's visit helps the practitioner understand the significance of the patient's symptomatology and evaluate its severity.

SICKNESS IS OFTEN TRIGGERED BY PSYCHOLOGICAL OR SOCIAL STRESS

The list of psychological factors that may precipitate illness is extensive. McWhinney[1] has devised a taxonomy that identifies seven general areas:

1. Loss: either personal, such as bereavement or divorce, or loss of something valued, such as a home, position, or object

2. Conflict: interpersonal or intrapersonal, having to do with conflicting internal demands
3. Change: triggered by either life cycle events or a geographical event
4. Maladjustment: interpersonal problems not having to do with acute conflicts; failure to adjust to occupational or home demands
5. Other stresses, acute or chronic
6. General isolation
7. Failure or frustrated expectations

We would add to this list:

8. Any anniversary of a significant loss or traumatic event[2-4]

These are the types of situations that impact the health of the patient. They are also the situations that lower the patient's threshold of tolerance for the discomfort of symptoms or the threshold for anxiety about symptoms. Since patients are often not aware of this relationship, they are very relieved when the practitioner helps them to make this connection. According to McWhinney,[5] sometimes the aim of therapy may not be to remove the symptoms but to help the patient to live with them.

STRESS OFTEN EXACERBATES CHRONIC CONDITIONS

A person whose diabetes has been well controlled for years may suddenly present in the office because of an increased blood sugar determined by home glucose monitoring. Perhaps the most important question that the practitioner can ask is "What is going on in your life?" It may turn out that the patient is afraid of getting fired, his wife is threatening to leave him, a teenage daughter has an older boyfriend who is making sexual demands on her, or perhaps there are financial problems related to college costs for children. These or any other situational stresses can easily precipitate an exacerbation of the diabetes and can best be managed with a psychological rather than chemical intervention.

Diabetes is not the only chronic condition affected by stress. Consider the following case related by one of our colleagues:

A 33-year-old female came to see me with a chief complaint of difficulty breathing. She reported a 2-day history of shortness of breath, especially with exertion, and a need for increased use of her albuterol inhaler. Other than a history of mild to moderate asthma, she has no significant medical problems. Her asthma occasionally flares up with seasonal changes, allergies, and strenuous exercise, but it is easily controlled with inhalers. She is married and has two young children. She works full-time outside the home. She reported no other symptoms, such as cough, sore throat, rhinorrhea, sneezing, fever, nausea, vomiting, or rash. Her allergies were well controlled with 10 mg of loratadine (Claritin) daily.

At this particular visit, the patient appeared fatigued and anxious. As I asked her questions about her breathing and other symptoms, she tried to minimize her disease and stated she just wanted renewals for her inhalers. At this point I decided to *BATHE* the patient. When asked what was happening in her life, she relaxed somewhat and offered a litany of stressful events that had occurred in the past several days culminating in a major screaming match with one of her children. When I asked how she felt about this situation, she replied, "And in the middle of it all, I just started wheezing!" She went on to say that she was feeling overwhelmed and that what troubled her the most was that her asthma was slowing her down and preventing her from addressing her family's needs in a timely fashion. I provided empathy and then we discussed ways in which she could cope, which included changing her inhaler regimen, stress management techniques, time management, and enlisting the help of her husband. She left the office appearing more relaxed and breathing easier.

THE PRACTITIONER'S INTEREST IS SUPPORTIVE

The practitioner's interest in the patient as a person is demonstrated by the inquiry about the social context of his or her problem. In this way, the practitioner demonstrates warmth and caring and affirms the individuality and importance of the patient. The patient has to make sense out of the practitioner's show of interest. One explanation is that the practitioner is a warm and caring person. This makes the patient feel safe and in good hands. Another explanation is that the patient is a worthwhile person who has some significance for the practitioner. This also makes the patient feel good. In either case, the patient will feel supported and hence be able to tolerate symptoms better.[6]

When practitioners routinely inquire into the circumstances of a patient's life, the patient becomes aware of the physical-psychological interaction. Understanding the effects of stress on the physical responses of the body helps to make the patient feel more in control and therefore less anxious. Becoming aware of the effects of stress is a prerequisite for learning to manage it. One of our faculty members related the following case of a 36-year-old divorced social worker currently living with a "significant other":

> F.L. presented with severe stomach cramps and wondered if she had ovarian cancer. A quick *BATHE* revealed high stress at work, which may also have accounted for her slightly low white blood cell count and elevated cholesterol. During the follow-up phone call to discuss the test results, the patient suddenly volunteered that she only gets the stomach cramps when there is high stress at work.

If we are not aware that we are becoming tense, there is no behavioral cue for applying relaxation techniques, be they physical or cognitive. Precipitants of stress are not always directly connected to the current situation. Understanding the significance of an anniversary, its potential for precipitating illness, and the high correlation of anniversaries with accidents[2,3] can keep patients from overreacting, turning acute events into chronic conditions, and setting unrealistic expectations for themselves.

A patient will almost sheepishly present with chest pain on the anniversary of his father's heart attack, saying "I know it's probably psychosomatic, Doc, but check it out anyway and relieve my anxiety. Every year at this time, I seem to develop these symptoms." After ruling out the acute condition and reassuring the patient, it is appropriate to encourage the patient to reassess his relationship with his father. If he has not completely dealt with his grief, it is important for him to focus on both the good and bad memories of his youth and come to terms with his remaining ambivalent feelings. This can be accomplished by writing about his father and their relationship, as we described in the previous chapter.

ELICITING PATIENTS' REACTIONS

Once the practitioner has determined the context of the visit in terms of what is going on in the patient's life, it is important to inquire about the patient's emotional reaction. "How do you feel about that?" is the most efficient question to ask, rather than "Why do you think this is happening?" or "What does your wife think about it?" The point is to get the patient to make an affective response. "How do you feel about it?" usually prompts a response that starts with "I feel. . . ." If the patient starts to offer other information or use the word "that" followed by a judgment, it is important for the practitioner to interrupt and to persist, "Yes, I understand, but how does it make you feel?" We would caution practitioners not to get caught up in the details of the patient's situation. Finding out who said what to whom has no therapeutic significance.

Our goal for the patient is to label and express feelings, giving us the opportunity to empathize. Then we attempt to focus the patient on a problem-solving strategy. Often, patients may admit to feeling anxious or depressed. Just having the patient acknowledge, "I am angry," or "I am sad," or "I feel rejected," "scared," "powerless," "overwhelmed," or "totally confused" is useful. Most people react automatically or semiautomatically to most of the events in their lives without any conscious awareness or thought about what they are feeling. When we focus their attention on their current affective experience, we break the pattern. When feelings are experienced, accepted, and acknowledged, they do not need to become psychosomatic symptoms. This is the essence of an effective psychotherapeutic intervention.

TEACHING A PROCESS

When the practitioner inquires about how the patient is feeling about a specific situation, the focus changes from what is happening to how the patient is reacting. This models a process that puts the emphasis on the patient's reactions while demonstrating the practitioner's concern. The clinician extends an invitation to get at the root of what is actually troubling the patient. Some patients have extreme difficulty in identifying or labeling their feelings. Their stories will focus on what happened and what they did or other people did in response. In this case the practitioner can use active listening as a way to focus on the affective domain: "Sounds like you were surprised and hurt when your request was denied." When this is acknowledged, it is important to follow up by asking "What about it troubled you the most?"

By inquiring about the significance of the event, the practitioner in a subtle way implies that the interpretation about what is troubling the patient is not necessarily obvious. This simple device may prepare the patient to see the situation as less catastrophic than had been assumed. It may also help the patient to recognize the need to develop potential solutions. The practitioner implies no meaning or judgment. The same situation has different significance for different people. The nonjudgmental nature of the practitioner's response makes the patient feel accepted and creates the conditions necessary to promote psychological change.[7]

As part of the initial inquiry, the practitioner now has a choice. One option is to ask the patient how the situation is being handled and then make an empathic response. The other option is to first acknowledge that the situation must be difficult and then to ask how the patient might handle it.

Many practitioners schedule patients with emotional problems for the end of the day in order to leave time to explore the situation fully. We strongly recommend against this practice, since it involves too much of an investment of valuable time on the part of the practitioner, creates unrealistic expectations on the part of the patient, and may not necessarily result in increased therapeutic benefits. Given a positive doctor-patient relationship, little difference in outcome has been found among psychotherapeutic techniques.[8-10] We therefore strongly urge primary care practitioners to practice, overlearn (do them so often that they become automatic), and routinely use our techniques because they are effective and do not take much of the practitioner's time.

EDITING THE STORY

In Chapter 4 we defined psychotherapy as helping patients to edit their stories. It is clear that the stories we tell ourselves about who we are and of what we are capable define how we will function in the world and to what extent we will achieve our potential. In other words, the stories we generate create our reality. This view is based on the postmodern understanding that we interpret our experienced reality through a pair of conceptual glasses—glasses based on factors such as our personal goals, our past experiences, our values and attitudes, our body of knowledge, the nature of language, and our contemporary culture.[11] There is no way to observe the world as it really is with pure objectivity. This concept is very useful from a pragmatic therapeutic perspective. When we get the patient to accept a new story, we help him or her to create a new reality.

The Story Must Be Heard and Reflected Back With Empathy

Patients must be allowed to tell their stories. In order to make therapeutic interventions we first hear the patient's experience of pain, frustration, anxieties, and perceived limits. It is hoped that we can encourage patients to give us a brief synopsis rather than a multi-volume saga. That is one of the functions of the BATHE technique, but we cannot provide reassurance or remove impediments until we understand the patient's concerns. Using active listening and reflecting back the content of patients' concerns let patients know that they have been heard and understood. When this is followed by empathic responses, patients feel competent as well as connected to the practitioner. This is a highly therapeutic condition.

Challenging Limits

It is important to listen for the defining limits in the patient's narrative: the words "always," "never," "everyone," "no one," and "can't." These words help to define the patient as helpless. Filters that selectively process experience must be exposed before behavior can be changed. Absolutes must be challenged. One or two questions can help to clarify the situation: "You always make mistakes? You mean, you have never gotten anything right?" "Everyone is smarter than you?" "How many people have you tested?" "No one has ever supported you?" An appropriate response might be "I'm sorry, that must feel awful." (Translation: I support you.)

However, the most important intervention is in response to the phrase "I can't," a clue regarding a limited sense of self-efficacy. Given motivation, there are very few things that humans cannot accomplish. In every case, when patients complain that they cannot do something, the practitioner can respond with "You have not been able to do that until now."

The Amazing Power of the Word "Yet"

The word "yet" implies that something is about to happen or will happen in the future. It also implies that it is possible. When patients state that they cannot do something, they are basing that assertion on past experience. When practitioners respond that patients have not been able to do it "yet," the implication is that the practitioner expects the patient to be able to accomplish whatever it is in the future. That is a powerful suggestion coming from a highly influential person. It challenges the patient's story and potentiates change. It is important for the practitioner to make the statement with assurance (it is always true). Other phrases, such as "Up to now this has been difficult for you" or "Up until this time you haven't succeeded at this," are equally useful; but we like the word "yet." It is short and to the point, and when you use it: You Empower Them.

Listening for limits highlighted by patients' statements about what they cannot do and responding with a counter statement that they "just haven't yet" constitute a very practical therapeutic intervention. When the patient returns for the next visit, it is likely that he or she will state that whatever it was has not been accomplished *yet*, but. . . . The practitioner will know that the message has been heard and is being processed. Change will follow. The patient's story has been successfully edited.

THE IMPORTANCE OF STRUCTURE

Ordinarily, when a practitioner invites a patient to talk without structuring the interview, it is possible that the patient will gain some benefit, but it can be a process that is quite random. In our experience patients will complain incessantly and repeatedly about the behavior of other people and circumstances that cannot be changed, thereby reinforcing their limited interpretation of their reality. Allowing patients to go on and on about these matters is countertherapeutic. It tries the patience of the practitioner and sets up unreasonable expectations, on the part of the patient, regarding the amount of time the practitioner has available. Also, often we find that the longer the patient talks, the more upset he or she gets. When recalling a litany of insults and injuries experienced, patients rekindle many negative feelings. By giving the patient valuable time and listening attentively to unchanging complaints, the practitioner supports the patient's distorted perceptions and the story remains unchanged. Ultimately, the practitioner may decide that it is not worth trying to treat the psychological aspects of a patient's problems.

Perhaps, over time, the uncritical attention of the practitioner may enhance the patient's self-esteem. This is the major assumption behind Rogers's client-centered therapy.[7] However, we have found that rather than letting patients continue to retell the same story, the more effective and economical strategy in terms of time and emotional energy is to briefly summarize, give an empathic response, and then make one or two interventions that challenge or potentially change patients' behavior or assumptive world view, as in the following example:

A 55-year-old woman comes to the office complaining of fatigue. She says that she has been tired for weeks. She has had no physical exam for years. There is no significant medical history. Asked about what is going on in her life, she says that both she and her husband work full-time, she is also a homemaker, and she takes care of her 17-year-old son, who is legally blind but has just been accepted into college. She looks frightened, depressed, and essentially closed. Asked how she feels about what is going on, she only volunteers that she is tired. The physical exam is unremarkable; blood and urine tests and a pelvic exam all are normal. The practitioner thinks that the patient might be depressed. He asks, "Do you have any idea what you might be depressed about?" The patient replies, "Depressed? I don't know if I'm depressed. I know I'm tired. I work a 40-hour week. Keep my own house. Cook dinner every night. I have a nice husband who would be happy with a bologna sandwich but wouldn't make it for himself." She pauses and then says, "Oh yes, my sister cares for our 90-year-old father. I go over there every Saturday to help out. I really wish she'd put him in a nursing home, but I feel guilty when I think that, and my sister won't hear of it."

The practitioner (challenging the view that wishing to put the father into a nursing home is any cause for feeling guilty) responds that he thinks that that is a perfectly reasonable way to feel. The patient sighs. She looks relieved and volunteers that she has done nothing for herself in recent times. The practitioner suggests that she make just one small change. The patient smiles, "I can do that. Thank you so much, Doctor, I feel so much better."

As we have said previously, the therapeutic intervention consists of interrupting fixed patterns of behavior and thought by focusing attention either on the behavior or away from it (distracting the person and/or focusing on other options). By *BATHEing* the patient, we are focusing on feelings, on interpretations, and on the behavioral responses of the patient and setting the stage for change.

Frequently the initial sequence is all that is required in the way of psychological support. It often helps the patient to gain insight into the particular situation and make a plan for resolution. It is only with those patients whose situational stress is currently unmanageable that one needs to engage in a specific therapeutic contract.

Fielding Unexpected Reactions During the Interview

Often as part of taking a history, a routine question about previous hospitalizations, family illness, or previous geographical moves may elicit a strong emotional reaction in a patient, that is, trigger painful memories. The practitioner may be at a loss whether to ignore, soothe, or deeply explore the reaction. *BATHE*ing provides a constructive alternative:

A young woman presented in the office complaining of a sore throat. Initial inquiry was unremarkable. However, when asked if there was any family history of rheumatic fever, she suddenly started to cry and recalled that while she was in high school she had been put to bed for several months because of rheumatic fever. The practitioner was first taken aback and hesitant to get into an old painful experience. However, since something had to be done, the practitioner decided to apply the BATHE technique. The physician inquired about the background, "You were in high school, about what grade?"

"I was just starting my senior year."

Going right to affect, the physician inquired, "And they put you on complete bed rest, how did you feel about that?"

The patient replied, "I felt so isolated and out of it."

The physician did not allow herself to explore these feelings further but inquired directly about trouble, "What about the situation troubled you the most?"

"I was afraid that I would not graduate with my class."

"How did you handle that?" was the final question.

"Well, there wasn't much I could do. I had to go to summer school. It was awful."

The empathic response followed, "I can see that that was a very difficult time for you. Tell me, any other serious illnesses?"

The patient responded, "No." Then after a pause, "You know, at this point it really doesn't make any difference. As a matter of fact, now that I think of it, I think I did better in college because I worked for a year first."

The physician responded, "I'm glad. Now I'd like to examine you and make sure that everything else is O.K."

FOCUSING ON OPTIONS

In dealing with a patient's situational stress, it is crucial that the practitioner not take responsibility for solving the patient's problems. In *The House of God*,[12] a biting satire about medical education, one of the primary truths (rule four) clearly states, "The patient is the one with the disease." If the patient is the one with the disease or the problem, the patient has a right to decide what, if anything, should be done about it. The practitioner has the opportunity to intervene in the process by simply making the patient aware that there are options and encouraging the patient to make a conscious choice about what to do. There are three useful strategies that can be presented to a patient: looking at the consequences, applying tincture of time, and choosing not to choose.

Looking at Consequences

The practitioner can encourage the patient to think about and/or list several possible courses of behavior and to sort out the consequences inherent in these choices. A good structure is to ask the patient to specify what the best and worst possible outcomes might be. Patients who are very angry often talk about wanting to kill the offending party. Rather than responding, "You don't mean that!" (Yes, they do, at least for the moment.) or "You can't do that!" (Yes, they can; it is not a good idea, but it is possible and unfortunately happens every day.), the effective reply is "I can understand that you would feel that way, but that does not sound like a very practical option when you consider the consequences. Do you agree? O.K. Let's talk again next week and see what you might do that's more practical." The implication here is that the feeling is legitimate (It is!) but that once the patient thinks about it, other behavioral choices will appear. Also it is clear that the decision about what to do can be deferred at least until the following week. This relieves some pressure. The notion of "What is the worst thing that can happen if you do this?" is a very important one for the patient to explore. If the potential outcome is totally unacceptable, unless the probability of its occurring is definitely zero, the patient is advised not to consider that particular choice. These pragmatic instructions will help empower patients to view their circumstances more constructively.

Applying Tincture of Time

It is often true that the more important a decision is, the less information we have to base it on and the less time we take to make it. We put a deposit on a desirable house after one or two brief visits because if we do not act immediately, someone else will snap it up. Then we spend days choosing among shades of paint or wallpaper patterns.

Often a patient who is reacting emotionally to an event may feel impelled to make a decision. Having learned of her husband's unfaithfulness, a wife may feel she must either leave him immediately or have an affair herself. Neither of these options is likely to have a positive outcome. Instead, the practitioner encourages the patient to take time to sort out her feelings. Reacting to an acute loss involves an increased intensity of pain. This pain must be accepted and experienced fully. Ultimately it will lead to understanding and personal growth. The practitioner offers support and schedules an appointment to talk again. The implication is that tincture of time will provide relief.

Choosing Not to Choose

In a case where all apparent choices are unacceptable and the patient does not want to pick the lesser of the evils, the practitioner can instruct the patient that for the moment at least the best course of action may be to do nothing. Sometimes not all the important information is available to make an intelligent choice. The critical question to answer is now "What is the worst thing that can happen if you don't make a decision about this?" To choose not to choose is an option that many people never consider.

As we have said, psychological pain is something that must be felt but does not necessarily require a behavioral response. Often there is no need to act, especially if the pain is induced by the actions of another person over whom we have no control. In many cases, breaking a pattern by not acting in response to provocation by another shifts the balance of power. When I refuse to accept the conditions of a current relationship, it becomes the other person's problem to decide what to do. There are times that being "passive aggressive" really pays off. In general, when faced with several unacceptable choices, it is a good idea to make oneself comfortable while waiting for something to happen. It usually does.

THE EFFECTS OF SYMBOLISM

One of the more fascinating aspects of practicing primary care medicine is the opportunity to engage meaningfully with a variety of people. The specialist who treats limited organ systems is excited only by unusual manifestations of disease and the opportunity to diagnose rare cases. The primary care practitioner can be endlessly fascinated by the varied reactions that different individuals have to the same circumstances. The particular meaning that each of us attributes to an event (the story) determines our reaction, rather than the event proper. In every case where a person appears to be overreacting to a particular situation, we can assume that a symbolic meaning to that circumstance is triggering the patient's response, as shown by the following example:

Mr. Harris, a 28-year-old white male, presented in the emergency room with chest pain and difficulty breathing of sudden onset. He had no risk factors for heart disease, and examination, electrocardiogram, and enzyme studies were totally normal. The practitioner was aware that Mrs. Harris was due to deliver their first child momentarily and that the couple was extremely happy about the prospect of becoming parents. Arrangements were complete, and Mr. Harris had planned to stay with his wife during the delivery.

After reassuring the patient about the condition of his heart, the doctor inquired about what was currently happening. She was informed that the obstetrician had just told the couple that the baby was in breech position and that he had decided to do a cesarean delivery. At this point the patient started to cry. He revealed that he himself had been a breech delivery and that his mother had died in childbirth. He was sure that his wife would not survive. He had so wanted to be present at the birth but now could not face the prospect.

The practitioner was able to reassure him about the improvement in obstetrical procedures over the past 28 years and the relatively low risk associated with breech presentation when cesarean delivery is used. However, the physician did point out that it was perfectly O.K. to be concerned and scared. The patient was then able to connect his severe reaction to his own tragic birth circumstances rather than the current situation. The physician suggested that perhaps the patient needed to bring a support person to the hospital for himself. The following week, a proud father, gowned and masked, held his wife's hand in the operating room and watched his son take his first breath.

When helping a patient tie a particular reaction to its historical roots, the practitioner implies that the patient can break the pattern of response and reassess the significance of that situation in the present. Up to now, you may have had a particular intolerance to people's loud arguing because when you were a child your parents fought bitterly. Listening to them, you felt helpless and frightened because your security was threatened. Whenever you heard people arguing, you felt helpless and frightened just as you did then. If a practitioner were to ask you gently, "Are you really helpless now? As an adult, is your security threatened?", you would become aware of the change in your circumstances and learn to monitor your reaction to loud arguments and, thereby, effect a change.

The practitioner's brief inquiry about the historical roots of an event can have a profound effect on a patient's self-esteem, sense of control, feelings of self-efficacy, and assumptive world view. It is not necessary to explore the circumstances, distortions, or details in depth. It is only necessary to point out to the patient that there appears to be an inconsistency in the severity of the reaction in relation to the apparent face value of the event. Once patients are in touch with the original onset of the problem they can be asked to write an autobiography, keep a journal of current reactions, or compare memories with various living relatives in order to sort out the origins of some of their stories and troubling interpersonal reactions. Often this will promote constructive dialogue between patients and the significant persons in their lives. The important issue is that the patient is the one who must understand and ultimately change the reaction. The practitioner's view of the situation, regardless of how accurate, accomplishes nothing. As Shem has said, "The patient is the one with the disease."[12] The patient also is the one who must make the connections and change the responses.

FOCUSING THE PATIENT IN THE PRESENT

All reactions to current life stress are significantly affected by past experience. However, when engaging a patient in a brief therapy session, it is crucial to stress that regardless of a problem's origin or historical significance (fascinating as that may be), the past is past, and all we have to deal with is the present. Dwelling on past hurts is not useful: "Do you still resent your brother now, because your mother always favored him when you were kids? Really?" "Gee, I guess I do." "My guess is that your mother did the very best that she could. What would it take for you to forgive her?" The reality is that when we hold on to grudges or nurse our resentments, our bodies pay a price.[13] We make ourselves miserable and do not actually affect the people with whom we are angry. In the past several years the interest in the effects of forgiveness has grown exponenetially.[14] It is a process that can be taught, as discussed in Chapter 10.

Just as there is no benefit to obsessing about past hurts, assumptions made about the future are usually wrong and destructive. When a patient generalizes from a current unfavorable situation to speculate about a bleak outlook, the practitioner needs to challenge this distortion; for example, "I understand that your husband has left you and that you feel very hurt. However, it is not legitimate to assume that no one will ever love you again." "Yes, it is very painful to have your article rejected by the *AAI Journal*. You worked very hard on it and were sure it would be accepted. However, but that does not mean that *no one* will ever publish it." "You are feeling very unhappy right now, but that does not mean that you will never be happy again." When a patient says, "I *know* that such and such will happen because it always has," it is important to correct him or her by restating, "You assume that such and such will happen. What is it that you could possibly do to change that?"

It is important to encourage the patient to take one day at a time. If the patient is in extreme pain, it may be necessary to suggest taking it five minutes at a time. Then the patient is to acknowledge that accomplishment. Patients should also be cautioned that wallowing in their pain is not constructive. If occasionally they cannot resist the need to wallow, they may be given permission to do so, providing they limit wallowing to five-minute sessions. Patients really respond quite well to this type of instruction. It puts their pain into context and gives them a sense of control.

These edicts, stated with the authority of the practitioner, and with the attributed social power inherent in the role, help the patient reassess the resources that are available for dealing with current problems. The practitioner's encouragement to appraise reality in the present, rather than dwelling on the past, which cannot be changed, or the future, which cannot be predicted accurately, is very productive. Patients are generally depressed about the past and anxious about the future. When we focus them in the present and engage them in constructive problem solving rather than fight or flight behavior, they respond amazingly well.

THREE-STEP PROBLEM SOLVING

We have promoted several "cookbook" approaches to therapy because they provide a simple structure through which to trigger a practitioner's efforts to help patients. In Chapter 4 we introduced the PLISSIT structure to determine levels of intervention from simple permission giving, to limited information, specific suggestions, and finally, a contract for intensive therapy. In Chapter 6, and the current chapter, we have repeatedly preached about the benefits of *BATHE*ing the patient to determine and manage the situational context of the patient visit. Now we propose a three-step sequence of questions that can be effectively applied to any disturbing situation. These questions are as follows:

1. What am I feeling?
2. What do I want?
3. What can I do about it?

This is often a useful framework for practitioners to apply to their own reactions, as will be discussed in Chapter 11. For the present, let us focus back on the patient. The series of questions now becomes the following:

1. What are you feeling? (Label the actual feeling.)
2. What do you want? (Specifically state your goal.)
3. What can you do about it? (Focus on what you can control.)

For example, patient X is complaining about how his daughter's attitude disturbs him. The practitioner asks, "What are you feeling?" The patient may try to continue ranting about his daughter's behavior and give examples to illustrate that she is not acting the way she should be. He says they fight all the time and he screams at her. The practitioner persists, "What do you feel in that situation?" or "How do you *feel* about that?"

It may turn out that the patient feels angry, hurt, frightened, discounted, disappointed, devalued, disgusted, or some other unpleasant sensation depending on the meaning of his daughter's attitude for him.

At this point the practitioner acknowledges that feeling and asks, "What do you want?" At first the patient will respond that he does not want to be in this situation and he does not want his daughter to treat him this way. The practitioner persists, "What do *you* want?"

"I want her to change her behavior." (Sometimes patients say they do not really know, in which case the practitioner can encourage them to think about that and come back to talk again.)

The final question is "What can you do about that? I understand that fighting with her has not been helpful." The patient may decide that he can reward appropriate behavior, discuss it quietly, present the situation to his daughter as a problem to be solved, negotiate a contract, and let his daughter know that he truly loves and accepts her. Sometimes there is nothing that can be done. Once that becomes clear, what the patient feels about the situation changes to appropriate sadness. It is hard to accept the fact that we cannot control other people's attitudes and behavior.

In any case, this three-step process is a powerful therapeutic intervention because it labels feelings, clarifies what the patient wants, and points to a direction for achieving these goals. It is economical in time and direct in therapeutic value, since it encourages new ways of thinking and behaving while discouraging the passive role. It also teaches the patient a strategy that can be applied to any number of situations.

PUTTING THE PATIENT BACK IN CONTROL

We have said that the feeling of being overwhelmed is generally the trigger for patients' help-seeking behavior. When the practitioner engages patients in problem solving, patients become aware that they have some control over the circumstances of their lives. Since the relationship with the practitioner is an ongoing one, patients sense that they have a partner and therefore feel less isolated. Someone cares and wants to follow their progress. If feelings of abandonment helped to trigger unpleasant reactions, now there is an assurance of ongoing support that will continue to be available over time.

The second important factor concerns patients' reactions to practitioners' expectations that they are capable of handling their situations. The practitioner clearly indicates to patients that their reactions are legitimate but that they have choices and that there are always actions available to them that will improve their current circumstances if only slightly. If a patient is able to hear and accept these messages, it will change how the patient feels about his or her ability to cope. Certainly the patient is not helpless and will no longer feel hopeless. This change in reaction may even make the situation appear less difficult and ultimately improve it. Consider the following case described by one of our graduates:

A 37-year-old, divorced, Egyptian female returned to the office for a follow-up visit for her elevated cholesterol and for her annual gynecological exam. She appeared particularly sad today; she did not smile, and she spoke with a monotone voice. It was more difficult than usual to engage her in conversation. On review of systems, she had multiple somatic complaints, such as lower back pain, shoulder pain, and headaches. She also had several neurovegetative complaints: 12-pound weight gain in three to four months, lack of energy, fatigue, difficulty concentrating, and difficulty falling asleep. I was concerned that she was clinically depressed.

When I asked what was happening in her life at that time, she admitted that she felt a great deal of stress because of overwhelming responsibilities. She admitted that she worried too much and that she knew many of her symptoms might be related to her worries. She is a single mother of two teenage girls; she works full-time and attends school part-time at the local community college. When asked what troubled her the most, she admitted that her husband deserted her and their children, leaving them here in the United States with her relatives, while he returned to Egypt with another woman and subsequently filed for divorce. She felt sad, angry, and bitter over these events.

When I asked how she was handling all this stress, she thought about it for a few seconds, and then her affect brightened as she replied that she normally maintains a positive outlook on life. She stated that her faith in God, and what He has in store for us, carries her through each difficult day. She also said that she is blessed to have multiple, strong family supports here in this country. The patient appeared quite relieved and justified when I empathized with her and pointed out that she was doing a great job holding herself and her family together, despite such adversity. The patient left the office smiling and thanking me for giving her permission to feel and express her emotions.

A constructive response to the practitioner's intervention will engage a positive cycle. We are all familiar with vicious cycles and downward spirals. Positive cycles are equally self-generating. When patients cease to feel overwhelmed, they resume their normal and more effective functioning. Mature coping mechanisms again become available. The patient's view of the situation broadens, and novel stimuli can be experienced and processed. This will lead to more effective problem solving and a better sense of being in control. This improved functioning will then be reinforced by success in achieving desired outcomes.

Focus on Strengths

Every person or situation has both good and bad potential. It is definitely more therapeutic to focus on positive aspects of a situation and on the positive qualities of a person. A glass that is half-full is to be preferred over one that is half-empty. There is strong evidence to support the need to be optimistic and to speak in positive terms. A classic study showed that patients react much more favorably to being told that there is a 68% survival rate than that there is a 32% mortality rate.[15] Common sense tells us these statistics are the same. We can only speculate that in the first instance a patient focuses on the word "survival" and in the second only "mortality" is heard. The numbers are discounted.

It is important to keep in mind that in every case, our patients have definitively demonstrated their ability to survive, since if they had not, they would not be appearing in our offices at this time. One way or the other, patients have surmounted the many challenges that are part of living in our rapidly changing society. We need to remember Theodore Rubin's insight that "the problem is not that there are problems. The problem is expecting otherwise and thinking that having problems is a problem."[16] It is how we react that matters. Once refocused on their healthy resources, patients will manage their problems and their lives in remarkably competent ways.

The Patient Is Responsible

Although the practitioner is available for help and support, responsibility for resolving the problem remains with the patient. The practitioner assumes the role of coach while the patient is the player who is held accountable for applying the strategies that have been discussed and for investigating various options. The practitioner expresses confidence in the patient's ability to gather and apply the resources necessary to arrive at a positive outcome. The patient is encouraged to stay in the "here and now," since fretting about the past or worrying about the future is not constructive. Things need to be taken one day at a time until there is some clear resolution. There is a mutual understanding that the situation will be discussed further at the next visit. The practitioner is interested in following all the developments. The time interval is clearly specified: "I want to see you next week and we will talk more." Although this approach works very well in many cases, patients do not always follow through as directed. Practitioners need not become frustrated. Instead we recommend applying the new scoring system and then redirecting the patient toward the desired goal.

The New Scoring System

In evaluating patients' progress, we recommend applying an innovative scoring system for tracking new behavior. In the best behavioral tradition, it is designed to focus only on positive changes and ignore lapses and can be expected to produce excellent results.

Since it has long been known that under stress people regress and are not able to apply most recently learned behavior,[17] lapses are to be ignored. Instead, patients are instructed to keep track of every time they engage in any new behavior. We are not interested in having them record failures (too many patients are stuck in their failure image), only instances of success. Patients are to give themselves credit (two points) every time they become aware of reacting, thinking, behaving, planning, or doing anything in a new way, that is, changing an old pattern.

Because it is hard to act in new ways or apply new behavioral techniques, doing it and recognizing doing it deserve two points. Patients must be informed that under stress it is normal and expected to react in old automatic ways. Certain behaviors have been overlearned and become a habit. Breaking habits is very difficult. The first and essential step to changing habitual behavior is to become aware that it is happening. Instructing patients not to get angry or abusive with themselves when they become aware that they have just reacted in an old way is the most important feature of the new scoring system. On the contrary, they get credit (one point) just for the recognition. One point is assigned for every time they notice that they have not taken advantage of an opportunity to react in a new way. Since this is scored as a success, it will provide motivation to apply the new behavior at the next opportunity. That is the reason for suggesting that patients give themselves credit (one point) every time they catch themselves doing something the old way.

Becoming conscious of behavior as it is occurring, starting to self-monitor, is a prerequisite for making lasting changes. By suggesting that the patient is doing something good (recognizing the behavior as it is happening), even when the patient is acting in the usual old way, we change the story. In this way we help patients to break the destructive cycle of feeling helpless and then abusing themselves for feeling that way. Instead, by changing the story before changing the target behavior, we put patients back in control, enhance their sense of self-efficacy, and induce positive change.

Chapter 8 will look at the content of the 15-minute therapy session and will introduce some further strategies and suggestions.

SUMMARY

Since illness or accidents exacerbate chronic conditions and sickness is often triggered by psychosocial stress, the practitioner should routinely ask all patients what is going on in their lives. The practitioner's interest indicates caring about the whole person. By making the inquiry routine, patients are educated to become aware of the interaction between their physical and psychological well-being.

If a patient is upset about the present situation, the practitioner extends an invitation to talk. The practitioner tries to establish the significance of the event for the patient and accepts the patient's feelings. When a patient unexpectedly reacts emotionally during the course of an interview, the practitioner briefly explores the issue by *BATHE*ing the patient. Patients' stories must be heard and reflected back with empathy, and then the limits must be challenged. By using the word "yet," the practitioner implies that the patient has the potential to change. In difficult situations, the practitioner suggests that there might be options, invites the patient to consider consequences related to different choices, and suggests that applying "tincture of time," or deciding not to decide, is a viable option.

The patient learns that events have a symbolic significance (which is different for all people), that certain feelings are triggered by old memories, and that self-esteem, the sense of control, and the sense of being lovable are all affected by the interpretations of historical events. The practitioner points out that these old interpretations can affect current relationships.

It is important not to generalize but to take life one day at a time. Patients generally feel guilty about the past and anxious about the future, but dwelling on past hurts is not useful and assumptions about the future are usually wrong, so focusing in the present and engaging in active problem solving are therapeutic.

A three-step approach to problem solving involves asking what the patient is feeling, what the patient wants, and what the patient can do to maximize getting what he or she wants. The practitioner's support makes the patient feel more in control. The patient has a partner. The practitioner indicates confidence in the patient's ability to handle things. The patient feels less overwhelmed and resumes functioning in a healthier mode.

The practitioner focuses on the patient's strength and acknowledges that the patient has survived similar situations, that support is available and can be asked for, and that the situation will be discussed further at the next visit. A scoring system that only records successes is instigated to reinforce new and more productive behavior.

REFERENCES

1. McWhinney, I.R. Beyond diagnosis: An approach to the integration of behavioral science and clinical medicine. *New England Journal of Medicine*, 1972, *287*, 384–387.
2. Bornstein, P.E., & Clayton, P. J. The anniversary reaction. *Diseases of the Nervous System*, 1972, *33*, 470–472.
3. Cavenar, J.O., Jr., Nash, J.I., & Maltbie, A.A. Anniversary reactions presenting as physical complaints. *Journal of Clinical Psychiatry*, 1978, *39*, 369–374.
4. Morgan, C.A., Hill, S., Fox, P., Kingham, P., & Southwick, S.M. Anniversary reactions in Gulf War veterans: A follow-up inquiry 6 years after the war. *American Journal of Psychiatry*, 1999, *156*(7), 1075–1079.
5. McWhinney, I.R. *A Textbook of Family Medicine*, 2nd ed. New York: Oxford University Press, 1997, p. 31.
6. House, J.S., Landis, KR., & Umberson, D. Social relationships and health. *Science*, 1988, *241*, 540–545.
7. Rogers, C.R. The necessary and sufficient conditions of therapeutic personality change. *Journal of Consulting Psychology*, 1957, *21*, 95–103.
8. Frank, J.D. Therapeutic components. In Myers, J.M. (ed.) *Cures by Psychotherapy: What Effects Change?* New York: Praeger, 1984.
9. Stiles, W.B., Shapiro, D.A., & Elliot, R. Are all psychotherapies equivalent? *American Psychologist*, 1986, *41*, 165–180.
10. Crits-Christoph, P. The efficacy of brief dynamic psychotherapy: A meta-analysis. *American Journal of Psychiatry*, 1992, *149*, 151–158.
11. Fishman, D.B. *The Case for Pragmatic Psychology*. New York: New York University Press, 1999, p. 5.
12. Shem, S. *The House of God*. New York: Dell Publishing, 1979.
13. Smith, T.W. Hostility and health: Current status of a psychosomatic hypothesis. *Health Psychology*, 1992, *11*, 139–150.
14. Enright, R.D., & North, J. *Exploring Forgiveness*. Madison, Wis.: University of Wisconsin Press, 1998.
15. McNeil, B.J., Pauker, S.G., Sox, H.C., & Tversky, A. On the elicitation of preferences for alternative therapies. *New England Journal of Medicine*, 1982, *306*, 1259–1262.
16. Quoted by Brian Baker. Quote of the day, 07/01/2001, http//:www.quoteworld.org
17. Cohen, S. Aftereffects of stress on human performance and social behavior: A review of research and theory. *Psychological Bulletin*, 1980, *88*, 82–108.

Agenda for the 15-Minute Counseling Session

What should transpire in the interaction between the practitioner and the patient in the sessions that are devoted primarily to counseling? That is the topic of this chapter. The objective is to promote change in the patient's behavioral, emotional, or cognitive reactions. In our view this can be defined as "psychotherapy," although we are acutely aware that both primary care practitioners and mental health professionals may be uncomfortable with this application of the term. From an interpersonal point of view, psychotherapy has been defined simply as "the systematic use of a human relationship for therapeutic purposes."[1] More recently psychotherapy has been defined not as a branch of behavioral science, but rather as a branch of rhetoric, the art of persuasion.[2] We can agree with this (see Chapter 3). In our view, when the therapeutic interaction with the practitioner is intended to affect the story patients tell themselves about the way things are and what is possible that can be defined as psychotherapy.

In contrast, to us, *counseling* suggests a process of giving advice related to a particular situation. It fosters dependency and implies that the practitioner has more insight into the situation than the patient does. We would like to propose a compromise: that the practitioner be aware of making therapeutic interventions but refer to the process as counseling. Jay Fidler, M.D., a renowned psychiatrist and teacher, once remarked that the primary difference between just playing with a child and play therapy was what went on in the therapist's head.[3]

As long as the practitioner recognizes that the objective of the 15 minutes spent with the patient is therapeutic change, it can be presented to the patient as counseling, which may make both the patient and the practitioner more comfortable. The patient is scheduled for one or more brief counseling sessions to talk about an ongoing situation that is causing emotional discomfort. We do urge the practitioner to interact with the patient with the awareness that the therapeutic process implies facilitating change in the patient's assumptions about the world and how the world can be accessed to provide more generously for the patient's needs. The practitioner's words and actions must be geared to promote the patient's sense of personal competence and connection to other people. The practitioner also intentionally supports strategies that help foster the patient's sense that the world is a reasonably reliable place. This is designed to impact the patient's sense of coherence, the factor cited as most significant in promoting health.[4,5]

Basically, the practitioner uses a variety of techniques to help the patient adapt to the environment in ways that will promote mental and physical health. Let us look at how all this can be effectively incorporated into a 15-minute counseling session.

THE OPENING INQUIRY

It is important to start every session with an open question and let the patient talk about whatever the patient has been planning to say, has been thinking about, or finds most important to discuss at this time.

"What has been happening since I saw you?" "Tell me how you've been doing." "What sort of things have you been thinking about since last week?" "Tell me how you've been feeling and what's been going on." Any of these are good openers. Then it is important to let the patient talk without interrupting for about two or three minutes. This gives the patient the opportunity to reflect on what seems to be most important currently. After about three minutes, it is critical to summarize what the patient has said in order to let him or her know that the practitioner has really been listening.

If the patient has not focused on events that have occurred since the previous visit, it is necessary to focus on the current situation and bypass elaborate background material. Asking "What is the most significant thing that's happened since I saw you last?" is a good way to direct the conversation.

Next the practitioner may assess the patient's affect and inquire by reflecting, "You look less tense, how do you feel about what's been going on?" or "How have you been feeling since I saw you last?" In cases where patients are out of touch with their feelings or have a hard time expressing them, it is useful to summarize the feelings that appear to be underlying the story. "Sounds like you are disappointed (or discouraged, frustrated, annoyed). Are you?" "I hear you blaming yourself, taking all the responsibility—do you feel guilty?"

Next, it is constructive to ask, "What is the worst thing that has happened since last time?" What has bothered the patient the most? It may be useful to explore what about the situation made it bothersome. It is the symbolic meaning of the event for the patient that is important. Finally, the practitioner asks how the patient feels about the way in which things were handled. An empathic response can be interjected whenever it seems appropriate.

It is also a good thing to focus on a success: "Tell me about one thing that you handled well or that you feel good about" or "What is the best thing that has happened since I saw you?" The small wins, and the sense of mastery that grows with effecting them, are very important.

The sequence of these questions is deliberate. If it sounds familiar, it should. It is the *BATHE* sequence. It focuses the patient in the present and helps him or her to identify and express feelings. It looks at what was most troubling (cognitive assessment) and the way in which things were handled (behavioral assessment). It helps the patient develop an awareness that both good and bad things happen during each time period and that the patient makes choices in responding to them. These techniques are generic therapeutic interventions. We are promoting them because they are useful and easy to remember and they work. They are certainly not the only way to do counseling, but they fit well into a brief-session framework and maximize the potential for positive outcome.

After going through the opening inquiry, it is important to make an empathic statement based on understanding the patient's experience during the intervening time since the last visit. If there was something positive to focus on, the practitioner might say, "I would think that you could feel very proud about having handled things in a new way."

If the patient has not been successful, a useful intervention could be "It must be really discouraging and painful when you are trying so hard to cooperate, that things at home don't seem any different. Still, you get points for having made some changes. What do you think you might modify more?"

REPORTING ON HOMEWORK ASSIGNMENTS

After the opening inquiry, focus shifts to the homework assignment. "Do you have the list of options that might be available to you?" "Did you talk to your wife and let her know exactly what is troubling you?" "What did you learn from keeping the log of all the times that you got very upset?" "What sources of support were you able to come up with?" "Tell me about the list of the positive and negative potential outcomes related to going into your own business at this time." If the assignment has been done, the practitioner takes this as a positive sign that the patient is exhibiting responsible behavior and is taking control. The session can then center on what has been learned from the assignment or on one thing about which the patient is most concerned.

If the assignment has not been completed, the practitioner must accept the fact. It is imperative that practitioners not scold or try to induce guilt in the patient. Therapeutic interventions provide new responses to old patterns. The practitioner simply states that for some reason the patient chose not to do the assignment at this time, adding that it might be useful to identify what obstacles were allowed to get in the way of doing the task and to recognize that there is always another opportunity:

"Mary, I can understand that you did not take the time to list the activities that really make you feel good. I wonder what makes it so hard for you to focus on things that you like. Do you want to do it for next week, or would you rather talk about it now?"

This approach communicates three important messages:
1. It is all right to be where you are. I accept you.
2. You are making choices that have some meaning for you.
3. However, there may be more constructive choices that you can make.

FACILITATING PATIENTS' ABILITY TO CHANGE

As we have said previously, people can and do make major changes in their behavior and in the way that they interpret the conditions of their lives (their story) but only when it is safe for them to do so and when they are ready. The brief counseling session can help to bring these positive conditions to pass.

Starting Where the Patient Is

The most important generic principle for making therapeutic interventions is that we have to start where the patient is (on his or her map). This is true in any type of teaching situation. In order to promote learning of any type, we first have to assess the level of the student's knowledge. If we were to present something that the student already knows, no learning would take place, since the student already has access to that information.[6] If we were to start at a level far more advanced than the student's background preparation, there would also be no learning because the new information would not be understood or incorporated.

If we are to be effective, we must start where any learner is at any given time. That means that we must accept our patients at their current levels of functioning, recognizing that as we do this without implied criticism, it facilitates patients' abilities to make small but positive changes.

Focusing the Patient in the Present

Since, by definition, we can only act in the present, we recommend that the patient generally be focused in the present. The only strong exception to this rule is the person who is working on a grief reaction and needs to review the history to sort out various feelings about the person, relationship, object, or position that has been or is about to be lost. We will say more about this in Chapter 9.

If a patient complains about how his mother treated him as a child, the practitioner can respond with some empathy but then wonder whether that is really relevant to how the patient presently treats his wife. What can the patient do to get more satisfaction from his current marriage? Also, what is it that the patient wants from his mother now?

Attentive Listening

Whenever the patient is speaking the practitioner should communicate interest and attention. This can be done by concentrating, maintaining eye contact, leaning toward the patient, refraining from writing, nodding approvingly, and responding at appropriate times. It is valuable to notice the patient's affect as positive or negative material is being related. If there is a discrepancy between the affect (facial expression and body language) and the content of the patient's story, this can be gently pointed out: "I notice that as you are telling me about all of the terrible things that are happening, you are smiling." This is important information for the patient to access. Perhaps he or she is just nervous, or perhaps this incongruent affect is a long-time problem and one of the reasons that the patient has difficulty with interpersonal relationships. Summarizing and reflecting back to the patient what has been heard and seen are useful, since they communicate that the practitioner has been paying attention and has understood. Consequently, the patient is able to move on and to make changes.

Probing for Feelings

Probably the most efficient therapeutic strategy is a two-step process of asking patients to identify feelings and then to accept these feelings as appropriate, given the underlying story.

When the patient relates what has been happening, good or bad, the practitioner inquires, "How did you feel about that?" It is interesting to observe reactions to this question. Patients often stop, look surprised at the direction of the conversation, and have to think for a moment before labeling the feeling. Many people are out of touch with their feelings, and most people are astonished when an authority figure expresses interest in their feelings. Often, patients do not respond with a label for a feeling but instead tell you what they thought or what someone else did. Let us look at an example:

Mr. Graham is relating how he asked his wife to make some changes in her schedule to accommodate him and that she agreed without giving him any argument.

Practitioner (breaking in): "How did you feel about that?"

Patient: "I thought she would just refuse to go along with me."

Practitioner: "I understand that, but how did it make you feel?"

Patient: "I was surprised and pleased."

Practitioner: "You really felt good."

In active listening it is useful to reflect understanding and acceptance by paraphrasing.

A patient has just related that he tried hard to get his wife to listen to how he felt about having to go to her mother's for dinner every Saturday night. Instead of responding, she simply gave him "one of her looks" and left the room.

Doctor: "So when Ethel walked away, how did you feel? Angry?" The patient nods.

Doctor: "I can understand that. You must have felt awful."

Giving patients permission to feel the feelings that have been aroused requires a minimal investment of time, energy, and understanding. A patient is overheard saying to her friend in the waiting room, "My doctor told me that my feelings are legitimate, even if other people see things differently or feel some other way." Her affect would have been appropriate for announcing that she had just won the lottery.

Acceptance Must Precede Change

Once having elicited and accepted the patient's feelings, if the practitioner thinks that it would be useful for the patient to become aware how his or her behavior contributed to creating a bad situation, then the next question might be "Tell me more about that. Then what did you decide to do?"

When asking for details or elaboration of events, we encourage focusing on the patient's behavior—what he or she thought and did and not stories about the thoughts and actions of other people. The underlying message is always that patients have choices. Indeed, they have power. Perhaps until now, the patient has not been aware of this.

Dealing With the Run-On Patient

Often patients find it difficult to stay within the structure prescribed by the practitioner. They will elaborate endlessly, or they will repeat themselves. When this occurs, it is essential that practitioners take a calming breath and then interrupt and summarize by saying,

"Yes, you told me about———. I know the details are important to you but tell me how it makes you *feel*." When patients talk about past events that cannot be changed, the practitioner should respond, "I hear how upset you are that things didn't work out. How does it make you feel *now*, and what might you do differently the next time?"

Getting patients to express guilt, anger, rage, or sadness helps them to accept their feelings and move on. Then they can examine options for dealing with matters now. They will become unstuck. Having escaped from the internal, stable, global explanatory box (see Chapter 4), they will feel less helpless.

Incorporating Medical Treatment

After the opening inquiry is completed, the practitioner may wish to follow up on any physical complaints. If there is an opportunity to "lay on hands," this is useful in helping the patient to connect physical and psychological symptoms. At this time, the practitioner may also discuss any changes in medications if they are part of the treatment. Medication is always an option to be used along with counseling, as discussed in Chapters 6 and 9. In the case of panic disorder,[7] generalized anxiety disorders,[8] depression,[9] and bulimia,[10] medication as an adjunct to cognitive types of psychotherapy has generally been shown to improve outcome. The written prescription should not, however, be seen as part of the ritual offering that the practitioner presents to the patient, as discussed in Chapter l. After the brief inquiry into the physical aspects, the practitioner focuses back on the psychosocial area: "All right, now let's talk about what you are going to do for next week."

COLLATERAL VISITS WITH FAMILY MEMBERS

As discussed in Chapter 3, one of the strong advantages the primary practitioner brings to the therapeutic encounter is the established relationship with the patient and the patient's family. A colleague, who is in solo private practice, reports the following case:

Gail, age 35, moved from Mississippi to New Jersey because of the demands of her husband's job. She is the daughter of alcoholic parents and has been suffering from an anxiety-depression syndrome for years. She has been treated with a variety of tranquilizers and antidepressants and is now struggling to adjust to life in a new community. Because of our inability to find a counselor with whom she felt comfortable, I, as her family practitioner, agreed to see her for some regular brief sessions. Some of her problems focused on the unresponsiveness of her husband, Jim. She felt that he would not want to come in but agreed to ask him. I had seen him several times, in the office, with the children and for problems of his own, and was confident I had sufficient rapport to enable us to talk freely.

I began the interview by saying that I understood that it was his wife who had asked for help but that I felt it was important at this time to elicit his support. During the introductory comments, Jim assured me that he felt that he had a good relationship with his wife, even though they did not communicate much. It took very little to make him happy. Knowing that his wife and children were provided for and having some peace and quiet for himself were all that he really needed. He realized that his wife needed more, such as a lovely home and an active social life. She also liked to be touched and caressed, but he was not "into" these things.

"How do you feel about these differences and the obvious lack of communication?" I asked.

He replied that he felt that they should improve their communication and, after some prompting, agreed that it was also probably important to their relationship to pay more attention to each other's interests but he "just hadn't thought much about it."

"For example," I asked, "what do you say when your wife says she wants to redecorate the dining room?"

"I tell her we don't have the money," he replied.

"Is that all?" I asked.

"Yes," he replied, "and the subject is dropped."

"Is there no way you could be more creative about this in order to satisfy your mutual interests?" I queried.

"Like what?" he wanted to know.

"For example, you might get a second job," I said.

"Or she might get a job," he replied quickly. This was something that Gail had wanted to do but was afraid her husband would not support. We agreed that this might solve several problems.

Moving on, I asked, "Do you remember your wife on Mother's Day?" (Knowing that he had this year.)

"Not usually," he said.

"How about birthdays?"

"Not usually. My family never made much of these things."

"How does she feel when you do remember her?" I asked.

"Oh, she loves it."

"Doesn't that give you pleasure also?" I wondered.

"Sure, but I just don't usually think about it."

"And in relation to sex, which you say you like, and touching, which you are not into, are you aware of some common differences between men and women in these areas?"

"Not really."

Here I mentioned some typical needs of women (often not understood by male partners) that were similar to those expressed by his wife. He seemed quite interested.

As we ended the interview (15 minutes exactly), he brightened up and said that this session had given him new ideas and much to think about and that he might be glad to talk with me again after he had time to do some homework.

In this case, the practitioner, by virtue of her established relationship with the family, in one visit was able to sensitize the husband to some very real problems experienced by his wife that under normal circumstances he would completely exclude from his map. The intervention proved to be extremely effective, and Gail's self-esteem increased dramatically as she experienced herself functioning well in her new job and having her husband act more attentive to her needs.

FORMATTING THE CHANGE PROCESS

Once patients recognize the need to change, it is useful to apply some easy to remember formulas to guide the process.

Behavioral Options

In general, it is good to focus on options for behavior. In Chapter 7 we introduced the following sequence:

1. What are you feeling?
2. What do you want?
3. What can *you* do about it?

This sequence helps to shift the responsibility for taking effective action to the patient. Rather than fretting about someone else's behavior over which they have no control, patients are encouraged to focus on novel approaches for getting their needs met. Inviting patients to respond to situations in a different way promotes new behavior. Breaking old destructive patterns is useful even if not successful at first. It demonstrates that there are alternative ways of behaving. If a wife cannot stop her husband from excess drinking, she can decide that since there is nothing that she can do to affect his behavior, she can change hers. She will stop arguing and fighting with him, stop aggravating herself about it, and engage instead in some activity that she enjoys. She may also decide to go to Al-Anon and get some support for herself. In this case, the patient has chosen an alternate way of responding to a situation. The situation has not changed, but her perception of it and her response to it have changed. As a result, she feels less overwhelmed. Moreover, since she has disturbed the homeostasis of the conflict in their relationship, the husband's behavior may ultimately also change.

Alternate Interpretations of Situations

Another useful approach is to encourage patients to find new ways to interpret situations, in other words, to change the story. Every difficult task can be viewed as an opportunity to gain skill and experience, to learn something of value, or to become stronger or more flexible. Seen in this light, the situation can prove more valuable and rewarding than had things worked out as originally desired or planned.

Patients need to learn that there are four healthy options for handling a bad situation:

1. Leaving it
2. Changing it
3. Accepting it as it is (and getting support elsewhere)
4. Reframing it (interpreting the situation differently)

Option 1

When considering leaving a situation, be it a relationship, job, or other intolerable circumstance, patients should be encouraged to assess what the best and worst possible outcomes might be should they leave. They can then be instructed to weigh the likelihood of each of these occurrences. Having a specific strategy to employ will give these patients a sense of competence and power in making the decision. If they decide to leave, they can be encouraged to plan the timing, obtain needed resources and other support, and practice what they want to say when informing the various affected parties. It is important that they consider contingency plans and explore all the relevant details. For instance, a patient with a chronic medical condition should think carefully about leaving a job and losing health insurance coverage without being certain that a new position will provide adequate benefits. This type of behavioral rehearsal fosters a high order of adaptive coping. These behavioral preparations, or potential scripts, constitute useful homework assignments, to be brought back to the practitioner for discussion.

Option 2

In considering whether a situation can be changed, patients need to look at what resources are available and what strategies might be employed. Has the patient communicated clearly with the powers-that-be regarding the level of dissatisfaction? Can the patient clearly define the problem and make suggestions for a positive resolution? Behavioral change on the part of the patient may ultimately change the responses of significant other people, thereby changing the situation. Sometimes outside pressure can be brought to bear on the situation, and often time alone will effect a change. In this case, it may be appropriate to accept the situation as it is for the moment.

Option 3

Accepting a situation as it is and not aggravating oneself by thinking about the fact that it should be different constitute a very constructive option. People make themselves miserable when they continually tell themselves the story that the circumstances they find are not as they should be. It is necessary to accept the fact that at any given time, things are the way they are. Given acceptance of that fact if, for instance, one's job is tedious, outside activities that are interesting and satisfying can be encouraged. Support groups, close friends, and exercise programs are all means of relieving stress. Taking pride in the quality of one's work and interactions with other people can also help to make accepting the situation more pleasant. Recognizing that time will probably bring change suggests making oneself comfortable while waiting for something to occur. It always does, although usually in unexpected ways.

Option 4

Changing the interpretation of a situation (i.e., reframing it or looking at it in a new way) is the most creative and satisfying way of dealing with difficult circumstances. When patients use novel ways of reinterpreting situations, when they change the story about the meaning of the circumstances, they are adapting in a growth-producing fashion and enhancing their mental and physical health.[11] It is the meaning that we attribute to a situation that determines how we feel about it, as shown by the following example:

Barbara D. was a patient with multiple problems, including severe back pain, generally unresponsive to treatment. She was moderately depressed and very concerned about her demanding husband and also about her mother-in-law, in whose home they lived. Barbara's treatment included 50 milligrams of amitriptyline at bedtime, referral to a biofeedback practitioner, and some assertiveness training. When Barbara complained that her husband "should not be so demanding," the practitioner suggested that this could be reframed to provide Barbara the opportunity to practice her assertiveness skills. The change in Barbara's attitude proved remarkable. She simply glowed the following week while reporting how she had handled several situations that previously would have left her feeling impotent rage. Not only that, but her back pain had almost entirely resolved.

THE PRACTITIONER'S ACCEPTANCE IS PART OF THE TREATMENT

In discussing stressful elements of the patient's life, the practitioner's attention and calm acceptance of the circumstances have a beneficial effect on the patient.

Accepting the Patient

The patient feels accepted as a person. The practitioner's interest is seen as supportive. Reflections by the practitioner help to make the patient feel competent. The patient feels valued, understood, and connected. The absence of criticism helps to counteract discouragement and self-doubt.

Accepting the Situation

By calmly accepting the situation, the practitioner becomes a role model for the patient. Together they look at a set of circumstances that, however unfortunate and difficult, first need to be accepted and then need to be handled. Just labeling the situation as a problem will change it. Problems lend themselves to a variety of solutions, some of which are better than others. There is now a direction for thinking constructively.

Accepting the Patient's Reaction

The practitioner's acceptance of the patient's reaction to the situation is therapeutic. Stating "This must be very difficult for you!" communicates to the patient that anyone would be stressed in similar circumstances. Usually it focuses the patient back on his or her strength: "Actually, I'm doing O.K., all things considered."

Assuming That There Are Options

Probably the most empowering aspect of the practitioner's approach is his or her assumption that options exist. We have talked a great deal in previous chapters about patients' assumptive world view, which is the story that they tell themselves about how the world operates. None of us experiences the world directly. Rather, we experience subjective representations of circumstances that we filter through our visual, auditory, tactile, or other senses and then interpret, based on our previous experience. We delete cues that do not fit into our previous frame of reference as though there were no such territory on our map. The resulting model of the world, the story that we create, determines what choices and limitations we think we have or that we impose on ourselves. When we mistake our limited representation of the world for the real world, we limit our options.

When the practitioner assumes that there are more options than patients are seeing (and it is not necessary for the practitioner to be able to generate them), patients begin to expand their models of the world, and their stories may allow for new interpretations. Patients start to include a variety of options and reexamine their limitations. The whole idea of the therapeutic intervention is to open patients up to existing possibilities and to invite them to look at their world, including themselves, in new ways. Patients become aware that they have choices.

Enhancing the Patient's Self-Esteem

Being open to possibilities is probably the hallmark of mental health. An impressive amount of data shows that positive illusions, rather than accurate contact with reality, lead to a sense of well-being and mental health characterized by the ability to care for others and do creative work.[12,13] As discussed previously, having a positive view of the self, an exaggerated belief in the ability to control the environment, and an optimistic view of the future is protective for mental and physical health. The practitioner's job is to help patients focus on positive aspects of themselves and their lives. When the patient expresses doubt about the ability to overcome some obstacle, the practitioner's confidence can be expressed by saying something like "You may have had problems with this in the past, but *I* see no reason that you cannot accomplish this now."

GIVING ADVICE

Practitioners are notorious for giving advice, and patients generally ask to be advised. They feel dependent, look up to the practitioner, and often want to be told what to do because they are afraid to make decisions or rely on their own abilities. Since they feel inadequate, they also feel out of control of their own destinies. Giving specific advice is always less effective than focusing patients back on their own resources, with appropriate instructions for developing alternatives. When the practitioner gives advice, the implication is that he or she has a better understanding of the patient's problems and options than the patient has. This does not empower patients. On the other hand, making patients aware of their own abilities and encouraging them to exercise their options are both therapeutic and practical. There are, however, certain suggestions that the practitioner can make. These focus primarily on the process of dealing with problems.

Behavioral Management of Children

Raising responsible children and enjoying the process require that parents develop specific skills. Not only in response to particular behavioral problems that parents relate, but also as part of well-child or routine visits, we encourage practitioners to support the following principles: rewarding good behavior and ignoring bad, setting strict limits on unacceptable behavior without making threats, using time-out to achieve control when children are uncooperative, allowing children to express feelings of all kinds but not allowing destructive behavior, and creating opportunities for children to make choices whenever possible.

Rewarding Good Behavior

When patients complain about their children's behavior, they can be instructed to apply behavioral principles. Primarily, this means reinforcing (rewarding) good behavior and extinguishing (ignoring) inappropriate behavior. Parents are encouraged to try to "catch" their children "doing something right"[14] and then to reward them. Patients must understand that attention is a reward, so acknowledging good behavior consistently instead of focusing attention on bad behavior promotes rapid improvement.

Setting Limits

Parents must learn to set strict limits on completely unacceptable or dangerous behavior. They must be instructed to be firm without making threats so that their children understand that the parents really mean what they say. When a parent says, "If you do such and such, I will punish you," it implies that the child has an option. The child has to decide whether doing the forbidden thing is worth the spanking, provided that Mother will follow through with the threat, which perhaps she will not. If, on the other hand, a clear statement is made, "I don't want you to do that," or "Stop that now!" there is no argument. In general, young children will try to please their parents. Limits must be set reasonably and enforced consistently. If necessary, parents can be instructed to remove a child from a situation physically, firmly but gently, and to instigate *time-out,* a respite in a boring place, as an effective form of discipline.

Using Time-Out

Anytime a child is out of control, not behaving according to set standards, or failing to respect another person's rights, time-out becomes a way to allow him or her to contain emotions without damaging the self or others. The child is escorted to a predetermined area (someplace considered "boring"—not the child's bedroom) that has a door that can be closed. The child is told that once he or she is quiet, back in control, and willing to cooperate, time-out will be suspended. Depending on the age of the child, two to fifteen minutes is usually sufficient to have the child calm down.

Expressing Feelings

It is essential that parents encourage children to express feelings but not to engage in destructive behavior, such as physical violence. Negative feelings must be allowed as well as positive ones. Children need to learn that becoming frustrated, angry, sad, confused, or cranky is part of the normal human experience. When children make statements such as "I hate you," this needs to be interpreted as "Right this instant, you are very angry with me." This can be followed with "I'm sorry that you feel this way, but in spite of the fact that you think it would be fun, I cannot allow you to . . . ." Children must learn that conflict is part of life but cannot be allowed to become physical.

Giving Children Choices

Parents must be encouraged to give children choices whenever possible. The opportunity to practice, from an early age, making decisions that impact one's life helps establish a positive sense of self-esteem and self-efficacy. For example, after a long day of shopping, one of our patients had a hard time getting a tired and cranky three-year-old to wash his hands before dinner until she asked him whether he would rather wash his hands in the sink or in the bath tub. He laughed, chose the tub, and immediately complied.

Dealing With Teenagers

Adolescents must be allowed to take part in making decisions that affect their lives and must also be held responsible for living up to their commitments. Parents should be encouraged to discuss reasonable limits with their teenage children and to negotiate joint agreements on acceptable rules. When a teenager does not follow through on a commitment, this must be addressed as a problem and renegotiated. In this way, the young person's self-esteem and self-control are fostered while the parent can relinquish the role of police officer.

Parents must be cautioned not to get into power struggles with their adolescent children. In a power struggle both parent and child lose, since when the parent wins the battle, the child's sense of control and self-esteem are compromised, generally leading to more destructive behavior. It is more constructive to jointly discuss options and to give the teenager an opportunity to decide among several acceptable alternatives. When parents treat teenagers as responsible individuals, express trust in their judgment, and respect their privacy, this information becomes part of the adolescents' sense of self, and they can be expected to act accordingly. Although it is foolish to minimize the dangers of peer pressure on teenagers to experiment with drugs and sex and engage in other risky behavior, what parents do to make their children feel wanted, included, valued, respected, and that they have social skills can help to protect them from engaging in self-destructive behavior.

Recommending Resources

Many useful books are available to help parents learn the above techniques. The classics, *Parent Effectiveness Training* by T. Gordon[15] and *How to Talk So Kids Will Listen & How to Listen So Kids Will Talk* by A. Faber and E. Mazlish,[16] are practical and effective. *The New Peoplemaking*, by Virginia Satir,[17] is a very readable and useful guide for managing children. All these are available in paperback. Parents can be encouraged to go to the library and browse or to look for paperbacks available in their local stores. The psychology/self-help sections of most bookstores have an incredible array of helpful, inexpensive manuals directed at specific problems. Relevant books can be read and discussed in subsequent sessions. The practitioner can save much time when patients get information from books and then come back to discuss their reactions. This is called *bibliotherapy*.[18] Appendix B lists helpful books that can be recommended to patients for this purpose.

Regardless of the recommendations made, it is important that the practitioner not forget to give the usual empathic support. "It must be very difficult to manage a teenager (three-year-old, two active children, or whatever) when you have all these other things going on in your life. Let's talk more about that next time."

Assertiveness Training

Patients should be encouraged to become appropriately assertive. In dealing with other people, patients must learn to see themselves and their desires as neither more nor less important than the desires of other people. Practitioners should advise patients to send "I" messages, learn to state their feelings, ask for what they want, and give their reactions to other people's behavior. For example: "When you ignore me when I walk into the room, I feel discounted" or "When I make dinner, and you don't come when I call you, I feel very angry." Saying "I don't like it when you don't do what you say you are going to do" is much more effective in getting another person to follow through on a promise than saying "You never do anything you say you are going to do!"

Patients must be counseled to persevere and insist that their rights be respected. Again, there are several books that the practitioner can recommend: *Your Perfect Right* by R.E. Alberti and M. Emmons[19] and *When I Say No, I Feel Guilty* by Manuel Smith[20] are outstanding examples. As before, the encouragement and interest coming from the practitioner are more important than reading self-help books. However, the support of the practitioner in conjunction with the outside reading is probably the most effective strategy.

Taking Care of Oneself

One prescription that we encourage the practitioner to give patients is the instruction to be kind to, to be gentle with, and to take good care of themselves. When patients are experiencing periods of high stress, they must be told to modify the demands they make on themselves. They cannot expect to function at optimal levels and will feel much better if they lower their expectations. Moreover, they can give themselves credit for dealing with a difficult situation.

Patients should be advised to give themselves treats, to take breaks, and to plan desirable activities on a regular basis so that they always have something to look forward to. It is important that they work on maintaining supportive relationships with people they enjoy and make the time to visit or at least keep in touch by phone. The message here is "You are important, and your happiness and sense of well-being are also important and must be a priority for you."

Patients should be encouraged to learn stress management techniques, such as controlled breathing, progressive relaxation, and meditation. They need to be encouraged to exercise regularly, choosing a modality they enjoy, and also need to learn to monitor and change their thinking patterns.

Distinguishing Among Thoughts, Feelings, and Behavior

It is important to teach patients to distinguish among thoughts, feelings, and behavior. Thoughts are constant internal messages that are often not noticed but are powerful enough to create our most intense emotions. We are constantly describing the world to ourselves (our stories) and comparing these descriptions of the way things are to the way we would like things to be. Based on these judgments, we then decide if things are good or bad, painful, dangerous, or just not as they should be.[21,22] These thoughts determine the way that we feel about a situation, another person, or ourselves.

Feelings constitute an automatic emotional response based on our judgments and interpretations. Feelings must be accepted, because they cannot be controlled directly. Given our interpretation of a situation (based on our story) we feel as we do. Cognitive therapy consists of challenging the underlying value judgments and assumptions that determine what we think. When we learn to modify our thought processes (i.e., edit our stories), moderate our expectations, and change our judgments, our feelings change.

Behavior is voluntary. We choose how we will act. When we are in touch with our feelings, we can learn to control our behavior. Our behavior is probably the only thing in life we really can control and should be aimed at getting us what we want and enabling us to present ourselves to the world as we wish to be seen. A practitioner can be very angry with a patient but keep the feeling hidden by choosing his or her words carefully in order not to intimidate the patient and to maximize the patient's cooperation.

In a brief counseling session the practitioner can help the patient to make distinctions among thoughts, feelings, and behavior; challenge irrational thoughts (the absolutes, unrealistic expectations, generalizations, and unfounded prognostications); accept feelings; and focus on behavior that can be changed.

Taking Responsibility for Our Feelings

The last bit of specific advice we suggest that practitioners offer patients is that it is useful to take responsibility for our own feelings. Few people realize that no one can actually make us feel anything. We feel the way we do as an automatic response to our interpretation of a given situation. A change in the interpretation changes the feeling. For example, if we presume that *all* practitioners reading this book will agree with our approach to therapy, we will feel very bad if some reviewers object to parts of the text or express reservations. On the other hand, if we hope simply that a few clinicians will find this book helpful and successfully use the techniques that we are proposing, we will be delighted when some people let us know that they are finding it useful.

Our current level of self-esteem, expectations for the future, and general outlook determine how we feel more acutely than what actually happens to us. It is the practitioner's task to make the patient aware that we make ourselves feel hurt, angry, frustrated, and rejected by the stories we tell ourselves about what has happened or is going to happen. The feelings we generate are often bad and painful. If we are going to turn off the pain, we must first become aware of what we are feeling, decide what about the situation is so troubling, and then modify those feelings by reinterpreting (revising the story of) our circumstances.

ENDING THE SESSION

Ending the session on time is important for both practitioner and patient. It is an affirmation of the patient's ability to cope and to apply the strategies discussed in the session.

It also ensures that the contract is valid and that the practitioner intends to follow through, thereby securing the sense of connection.

At the end of the allotted time, the practitioner should make an honest comment acknowledging a positive aspect of how the patient is dealing with the situation. It is helpful for the practitioner to express the feeling that it would be nice if there were more time (it lets the patient know that the practitioner values the contact) and that he or she is looking forward to continuing the discussion at the next scheduled session. The importance here is keeping the connection. The patient is instructed to call if something serious occurs in the meantime.

Homework

The specific homework task for the intervening time is jointly determined. The patient makes a contract with the practitioner agreeing to keep a journal, prioritize problems, find a specific book, engage in regular exercise, or in general monitor changes in behavior and the resultant consequences.

It is important that the time spent with the practitioner be devoted to building skills that the patient can use to change interactions with the significant others in his or her life. The visit with the practitioner provides direction and helps to make the patient aware of existing options and his or her power to put them into effect. It is up to the patient to chart his or her own progress during the intervening time. Homework assignments, particularly writing tasks, have been shown to be highly effective in promoting therapeutic change.[23-25] The process of doing the homework will be discussed at the next session. Knowing that the practitioner will be expecting a report helps motivate the patient to follow through on the assignment, as shown by the following example:

Carol G. is a 22-year-old white female and mother of two children (three and five years old) who is currently living with a boyfriend; she came to the office complaining of two weeks of dizziness. She seemed totally overwhelmed by the multiple problems in her life. For a homework assignment the practitioner suggested that Carol keep a journal and record all instances of dizziness and the particular circumstances when they occurred. Returning the following week, Carol was able to recognize that her dizziness occurred primarily when she felt most out of control, dealing with her estranged husband, her in-laws, her child's teacher, and her mother.

For the following week she was given the assignment to "do one thing nice for yourself." The resulting change was dramatic. Carol had decided to have lunch with a friend, leaving her mother to babysit. She and her friend talked through her problems and after sleeping soundly that night, Carol finally contacted a lawyer to start divorce proceedings.

Time Allocation

In general, the patient should be allowed to talk for 12 minutes out of the 15. Brief comments from the practitioner should keep the patient focused on one or two tasks that can be used as preparation for the next session. Dealing with only one or two issues during a particular session prevents the patient from becoming confused or overloaded. Thus the practitioner is teaching a process while treating a person.

Chapter 10 will look at some specific approaches to difficult patient encounters. We will provide some direction for treating the hypochondriacal patient, the grieving patient, the anxious or depressed patient, the suicidal patient, and the patient who must be referred because the practitioner feels uncomfortable. We will also discuss how these techniques can be applied to children.

Now let us look at a case that was handled by a young practitioner under our supervision and is typical of the effective outcome that can be expected over time:

Daniel G., a 16-year-old white male, presented at the Family Practice Center, on a Tuesday afternoon in late November, complaining of dizzy spells. The previous Sunday he had felt light-headed and dizzy and actually passed out. The patient said there had been two or three previous episodes but denied recent fever, palpitations, or chest pain.

Daniel and his mother had recently moved into the area to live with his grandmother. He related that he had no friends and was mostly interested in his baseball card collection. He admitted that he felt bad about the fact that he had no father and that his mother was crippled and confined to a wheelchair. The patient revealed that he wanted to become a carpenter.

A physical examination, including a complete neurological exam, was normal, allowing the practitioner, for the moment, to rule out an impending catastrophic medical event. His impression was vasovagal syncopal episodes. For completeness, routine laboratory tests were ordered, but the practitioner was more concerned that this patient needed emotional support. Daniel G. was a shy, sensitive individual with many emotional problems and no one to talk to. This made him feel very depressed. The practitioner made a contract for follow-up in one week with the expressed intention of seeing the patient for counseling.

In the course of having blood drawn, the patient became dizzy and his blood pressure dropped to 60/40, reinforcing the contention that this patient's symptoms were manifestations of vagal activity. In a half-hour his blood pressure had returned to normal, and the patient was released.

Daniel returned the following week. There had been no further episodes of dizziness. He then started to talk about his home situation. There was a horrendous history of abuse on the part of a man living with the mother and constant moves. The practitioner gave support and focused the patient on the present situation. Daniel had made a new friend in school and felt good about that, but he expressed a desire to transfer to vocational school. The practitioner said he would look into the possibility.

A contract was made to see the patient regularly once each week for 15-minute sessions. During the third session, Daniel appeared nervous and depressed. His affect was rather flat. He seemed to have nothing much to say. He wondered why the practitioner was interested in seeing him. The practitioner said that he enjoyed talking with Dan and would like to help him to learn to make other friends and focus on planning his life.

By the fourth week, the patient was much more cooperative. He was happy about a project in school and spontaneously started to share some of his interests. During Christmas week, the patient canceled his appointment. He arrived early in January complaining of a head cold but feeling much happier. It was during this session that the patient revealed a history of sexual abuse occurring several years previously and expressed how happy he was to be receiving counseling. The practitioner assured Daniel that it was not his fault that he had been abused and acknowledged that it must have been awful for him. This seemed to relieve the boy. The subject was brought up several weeks later but seemed to have lost its impact.

Over the next several months, Daniel was seen regularly for counseling every other week. In time, he became involved with the golf club at school and made one close friend. He was treated for a sore throat and some nose bleeds and developed a very relaxed and trusting relationship with his doctor. After about one year, his afternoon job prevented him from attending his sessions regularly. A sports physical clearing him for team participation is the last item in the chart. When Daniel moved away at 17½ years of age, he appeared to be a rather confident, reasonably well-adjusted young man who was clear about his goals and directed toward achieving them.

SUMMARY

The opening inquiry of a counseling session should focus on the present situation, a report on the homework assignment, and the best and worst things that transpired in the interim since the previous visit. The practitioner always starts where the patient is and communicates interest through attentive listening. Questions should generally probe for feelings and what the patient personally did in response to circumstances. Medication, laying-on of hands through examinations, and collateral visits with family members constitute other options that can be exercised.

In general, patients should be focused in the present. They are encouraged to focus on what they are feeling, what they want, and what they can do about it. Four healthy options for handling a painful situation are leaving it, changing it, accepting it with additional support, and reframing or reinterpreting (changing the story) it in a positive manner.

Practitioners must gently set limits on the amount of detail or repetition that a patient presents. The practitioner is supportive of the patient. The practitioner's acceptance is therapeutic. The practitioner accepts the patient, the situation, and the patient's reaction to the situation but assumes that there are always options that have yet to be considered.

In giving advice, the practitioner focuses on the process of dealing with problems, rather than their content. Advice may be given regarding behavioral strategies for managing children, becoming assertive, and taking care of the self. The practitioner points out the differences among thoughts, feelings, and behavior and how thoughts (judgments and/or stories) may be modified, with resulting emotional changes. Patients are held responsible for their own feelings. At the end of the session the practitioner extends the contract through the assignment of homework and the expectation that the patient will return to report on the accomplishment of a particular task. During the session the patient should speak about 12 minutes, with brief comments from the practitioner focusing on constructive elements. Time limits should be strictly adhered to. A successful counseling relationship with a teenager spanning over one year's time is described.

REFERENCES

1. Anchin, J.C., & Kiesler, D.J. *Handbook of Interpersonal Psychotherapy*. New York: Pergamon, 1982. Cited by Butler, S.F., & Strupp, H.H. Specific and nonspecific factors in psychotherapy: A problematic paradigm for psychotherapy research. *Psychotherapy*, 1986, 23, 36.

2. Fischer, A.R., Jome, L.M., & Atkinson, D.R. Reconceptualizing multicultural counseling: Universal healing conditions in a culturally specific context. *The Counseling Psychologist*, 1998, *26*, 525–588.

3. Fidler, J. Personal communication. Rutgers Community Mental Health Center Group Psychotherapy Training Program, 1974.

4. Antonovsky, A. *Health, Stress, and Coping*. San Francisco: Jossey-Bass, 1979.

5. Suominen, S., Helenius, H., Blomberg, H., Uutela, A., & Koskenvuo, M. Sense of coherence as a predictor of subjective state of health: Results of 4 years of follow-up of adults. *Journal of Psychosomatic Research*, 2001, *50*, 77–86.

6. Whitman, N.A., & Schwenk, T.L. *Preceptors as Teachers: A Guide to Clinical Teaching*. Salt Lake City, Utah: University of Utah School of Medicine Press, 1984.

7. Ballenger, J.C. Panic disorder in the medical setting. *Journal of Clinical Psychiatry*, 1997, *58*(suppl. 2), 13–17.

8. Power, K.G., Simpson, R.J., Swanson, V., & Wallace, L.A. Controlled comparison of pharmacological and psychological treatment of generalized anxiety disorder in primary care. *British Journal of General Practice*, 1990, *40*, 289–294.

9. Brown, C., Schulberg, H.C., & Prigerson, H.G. Factors associated with symptomatic improvement and recovery from major depression in primary care patients. *General Hospital Psychiatry*, 2000, *22*(4), 242–250.

10. Agras, W.S., Crow, S.J., Halmi, K.A., Mitchell, J.E., Wilson, G.T., & Kraemer, H.C. Outcome predictors for the cognitive-behavioral treatment of bulimia nervosa: Data from a multisite study. *American Journal of Psychiatry*, 2000, *157*, 1302–1308.

11. Vaillant, G.E. Natural history of male psychologic health: Effects of mental health on physical health. *New England Journal of Medicine*, 1979, *301*, 1249–1254.

12. Taylor, S.E., & Brown, J.D. Illusion and well-being: A social psychological perspective on mental health. *Psychological Bulletin*, 1988, *103*, 193–210.

13. Taylor, S.E., & Aspinwall, L.G. Mediating and moderating processes in psychosocial stress: Appraisal, coping, resistance and vulnerability. In Kaplan, H.B. (ed.) *Psychosocial Stress: Perspectives on Structure, Theory, Life Course, and Methods*. San Diego: Academic Press, 1996, pp. 71–110.

14. Blanchard, K., & Johnson, S. *The One Minute Manager*. New York: William Morrow & Co., 1982.

15. Gordon, T. *Parent Effectiveness Training: The Proven Program for Raising Responsible Children*. New York: Crown Publishing Group, 2000.

16. Faber, A., & Mazlish, E. *How to Talk So Kids Will Listen, How to Listen So Kids Will Talk*, 20th ed. New York: William Morrow & Co., 1999.

17. Satir, V. *The New Peoplemaking*. Palo Alto, Calif.: Science and Behavior Books, 1988.

18. Jamison, C., & Scogin, F. The outcome of cognitive bibliotherapy with depressed adults. *Journal of Consulting and Clinical Psychology*, 1995, *63*(4), 644–650.

19. Alberti, R.E., & Emmons, M. *Your Perfect Right*, 8th ed. San Luis Obispo, Calif.: Impact Publishers, 2001.

20. Smith, M.J. *When I Say No, I Feel Guilty*. New York: Bantam Press, 1975.

21. Beck, A.T. *Cognitive Therapy and Emotional Disorders*. New York: New American Library, 1979.

22. Ellis, A. *A New Guide to Rational Living*. North Hollywood, Calif.: Wilshire Books, 1975.

23. Cameron, L.D., & Nicholls, G. Expression of stressful experiences through writing: Effects of a self-regulation manipulation for pessimists and optimists. *Health Psychology*, 1998, *17*(1), 84–92.

24. Smyth, J.M., Stone, A.A., Hurewitz, A., & Kaell, A. Effects of writing about stressful experiences on symptom reduction in patients with asthma or rheumatoid arthritis: A randomized trial. *Journal of the American Medical Association*, 1999, *281*(14), 1304–1309.

25. Burns, D.D. Homework facilitates positive changes in depression. *Journal of Consulting and Clinical Psychology*, 2000, *68*, 46–56.

CHAPTER 9

Role of Pharmacotherapy

There is an important role for pharmacotherapy not as a substitute for but as an adjunct to psychological support, talk therapy, and other behavioral interventions in primary care practice. The dramatic increase in the use of psychotropic medications in the outpatient setting over the past 10 years supports practitioners' belief in their efficacy.[1] The combination of psychotherapy and pharmacotherapy often yields results that are clinically superior to either one alone.[2] We view the two as being complementary, not competitive or mutually exclusive.

The choice of what form of therapy to use for a particular patient is a matter of clinical judgment, but we hope to provide enough guidance in this text to help the clinician make a reasonable choice. However, this chapter is not meant to be an exhaustive pharmacopeia of agents available for the treatment of mental health disorders. Our goal is simply to increase the primary care practitioner's understanding of available pharmacotherapeutic agents in order to facilitate effective and appropriate prescribing.

Since we wish to approach this subject from a patient-centered perspective, we will be dealing with the application of pharmaceutical agents for various clinical diagnoses rather than listing them by their activity and pharmacological drug classification. It is our hope that this process will be clinically relevant. Our emphasis will be on those disorders amenable to psychopharmacological treatment in the primary care setting, such as anxiety, depression, attention-deficit/hyperactivity disorder, eating disorders, and Alzheimer's disease, since they are frequently encountered and have good therapeutic outcomes when managed comprehensively by an informed primary care practitioner.

ANXIETY AND DEPRESSIVE DISORDERS

Anxiety and depressive disorders are commonly encountered in our society and frequently occur concomitantly.[3] Indeed, pure anxiety or pure depression is the more unusual presentation.[4] Therefore, when making a diagnosis of a given patient, we must weigh whether the depressive symptoms or the anxiety symptoms are the more pervasive. Accordingly, it is useful to select a pharmaceutical agent that is appropriate for both conditions but perhaps is more effective for one than the other. Antidepressants are frequently employed here, because a number of them appear to benefit depressed patients also suffering from a broad spectrum of co-morbid anxiety disorders.[5-7] The following case illustrates this application:

M.A. is a 24-year-old single mother with one child, age six years. She was seen in the office complaining of being "tired all the time" of many months' duration. Her vital signs, included height and weight, were within normal limits and essentially unchanged from her last visit eight months previously. When she was asked by the clinician to expand on her symptoms all she could add was that she just didn't feel "very good" and was "dragging herself from place to place." She was then asked *what was going on in her life*, to which she responded, "Not very much. I live with my parents, and that is kind of boring, but it is also a necessity because my salary as a teacher's aide won't allow me to live on my own and still support my child." Asked *how she felt about that*, she responded, "I feel sort of hopeless because I'm young and yet I'm stuck with this situation." When asked *what troubled her the most* about the situation she related that "I'd love to be out from underneath the scrutiny of my parents. My mother makes me really nervous because she second-guesses everything I do and my father tries to tell me how to run my life. I guess they feel that it's their responsibility because I screwed up once and found myself in this situation." When asked *how she was handling this* she answered, "Not very well. I have a hard time sleeping, either falling asleep or waking up early in the morning. I am so jittery and jumpy, and I cry at the drop of a hat." She denied any suicidal ideation but did admit to feeling both hopeless and helpless; hopeless because of the situation she was in and helpless to do anything about it.

The clinician empathetically responded, saying that she understood that it must be very difficult to function well under these circumstances but that there may be some things the patient could do to improve her situation. She suggested that after the patient dressed they'd explore some of these possibilities together. The initial clinical impression was that this patient suffered mixed anxiety and depression but that depression was perhaps the more dominant symptom. Therefore, in addition to psychological support, she was given a pharmacotherapeutic agent that had both anti-depressant and anxiolytic actions.

Diagnosing and Treating Anxiety Disorders

Because anxiety is such a prevalent condition in our society, one needs to maintain a high index of suspicion regarding this disorder while obtaining a history. If in the process of *BATHE*ing the patient the clinician suspects that the patient may have an anxiety disorder, the SWIKIR Anxiety Scale can be employed to further refine the diagnostic process.[8] This scale assigns one point for each of the following complaints: (1) *S*omatic symptoms; (2) *W*orries; (3) *I*rritability; (4) *K*eyed up, on edge; (5) *I*nitial insomnia; and (6) *R*elaxation difficulties. Patients with a SWIKIR Anxiety Scale score of at least 3 are assumed to have a significant probability of a clinically important anxiety disorder.

If the clinician suspects that the patient has either an acute (DSM-IV adjustment disorder with anxiety) or generalized anxiety disorder, a number of effective anxiolytics can be employed in combination with behavioral or talk therapy. These newer anxiolytics, primarily in the benzodiazepine or the azaperone classes, have largely replaced the sedating barbiturates and meprobamate that had been mainstays of therapy in the past.

The benzodiazepines are effective agents, well studied, and frequently very beneficial if used regularly for relatively short periods of time (up to six weeks). Beyond that time frame there is some evidence that patients may begin to demonstrate symptoms of addiction and tolerance and experience adverse effects on attempts to withdraw the agent.[9] On the other hand, there also are studies purporting that these agents are seldom abused, particularly in persons who have no history of substance abuse.[10] As is usually the case, clinical judgment as to the risk/benefit ratio needs to be exercised before any pharmaceutical agent, including a benzodiazepine, is prescribed.

H.T., a 57-year-old accountant, was seen in the office suffering from extreme agitation and poor sleep. His wife, at her request, accompanied him. It was obvious that he was agitated and restless, and his wife seemed at a loss as to how to deal with him. After a few pleasantries he was asked directly *what was going on in his life*, and he blurted out that he had recently learned that he was to be *RIF*ed (reduction in force, i.e., let go) from a company for which he had been working for 35 years. His wife appeared shocked! He hurriedly went on to state that he had not known how to tell her about this because he knew she would be upset, particularly in view of all the sacrifices they had made for the company.

The balance of the *BATHE* inquiry revealed that he was obviously upset, unable to eat or sleep properly, and bothered by both the loss of his job and his inability to deal with it. At the same time, his wife, in tears, confessed that she was relieved that this was all it was. She had been afraid that he had learned he had some sort of terminal illness or other problem. She observed that they could get through this, since they have been able to overcome other obstacles in their life together. He seemed to be visibly relieved by both the attention from his physician and his wife's support.

However, he did volunteer that his jitteriness and jumpiness were interfering with his ability to function and think clearly. Therefore his clinician thought it was best that he be placed on short-term benzodiazepine therapy to calm him down and, in the process, enhance his coping skills. He was seen two weeks later, in a much-improved state of mind, and his wife related that both of them were working diligently to plan for the future. His benzodiazepines were tapered over the succeeding week, and the patient continued to do well. When last seen, he had made a complete adjustment and found part-time work that was even more to his liking than his former job!

The benzodiazepines are extremely effective agents for short-term use to improve the ability to function for patients in a crisis and to restore their ability to sleep.

Management of Chronic Anxiety Disorders

A recent study of chronic anxiety conditions treated in primary care found that cognitive and behavioral treatments whose effectiveness has been empirically validated were not as frequently used as would be desired.[11] Patients want that magic pill to make their symptoms go away.

Azaperone is effective for long-term treatment of generalized anxiety disorder (GAD) but require a period of titration to achieve effectiveness. This process may last as long as six weeks, and therefore azaperone is not indicated for the treatment of acute anxiety disorders (less than six weeks' duration).

J.R. was a 33-year-old single woman who presented to the office with a chief complaint of persistent headaches and insomnia, symptoms she had since she was a teenager. Although her symptoms had not gotten much worse over time, they had also not gotten better. She stated she was just "tired of not feeling well." She had seen other doctors for these problems from time to time, but none had helped her very much. She described her headaches as being dull in character, being located at the back of her neck, and occurring two or three times per week, usually toward the end of the workday. Her insomnia was characterized by an inability to get to sleep at least two or three nights per week. Typically she would just lie in bed and stare at the ceiling with her mind racing with thoughts about what happened during the day. She had recently been evaluated by a neurologist for the headaches and was told that "she didn't have a brain tumor," just "tension headaches." She was given an NSAID (nonsteroidal antiinflammatory drug) for her headaches. Although she was never formally treated for insomnia, she tried some over-the-counter sleep preparations but did not find them to be effective.

She had no significant past medical history other than the usual childhood illnesses. There was a family history of depression. Her brother took antidepressants, and her sister had episodes of postpartum depression following the birth of both her first and second child. The patient's father was a known alcohol abuser, and her mother had had problems with her "nerves," the exact nature of which was unclear to the patient. The patient was experiencing high levels of stress at work with escalating increases in her responsibilities and greater demands on her productivity. She admitted that she was drinking more lately to enable her to relax. When pressed further on this issue she confessed to drinking a glass or two of wine with her evening meal on workdays but not on weekends. Her *CAGE* screening questionnaire was negative for all four questions (Cut down, Annoyed, Guilt, Eye-opener).[12] Her physical examination, including a neurological examination, was within normal limits although she appeared jittery throughout the examination.

When asked about *what was going on in her life*, she admitted "not very much other than work" and she volunteered that perhaps if there were more things happening she would be less preoccupied with her symptoms. When *asked how she felt about that*, she replied that she was just getting more jittery and nervous and was afraid that this was beginning to affect her work and maybe ultimately her employment. When asked *what troubled her the most*, she responded that the symptoms were just going on and on and on with no end in sight. When asked *how she was handling that*, she admitted that she was afraid that she would start drinking more or lash out at her co-workers out of a sense of frustration.

Her physician empathized with her situation and then explained that her somatic symptoms were most likely the result of a condition known as generalized anxiety disorder that frequently produces this sort of symptomatology. He went to great lengths to reassure her that this was not a sign of weakness or moral failure but rather a treatable biochemical imbalance they could start working on immediately. The clinician suggested that she take an azaperone and they would titrate the dose over the first six weeks while they worked through various strategies to enable her to better cope with her generalized anxiety disorder. She was seen in the office on a weekly basis early on, then biweekly as her condition improved, and finally monthly over the course of a year. During this time she received psychological support as well as medication for the treatment of her anxiety. Eventually she learned stress management techniques and gained sufficient psychological insight so that her anxiolytics could be discontinued. She is still seen monthly by the clinician, has continued to do well, is relatively free of symptoms, and is a much happier individual.

TREATMENT OF OTHER ANXIETY DISORDERS

Since making a diagnosis is of paramount importance when prescribing medication, it may be useful to discuss some other disorders listed under "anxiety" in the DSM-IV, published by the American Psychiatric Association, that may be encountered by primary care practitioners.[13] These include specific phobias, obsessive-compulsive disorder (OCD), social phobia, posttraumatic stress disorder (PTSD), and panic disorder.

Obsessive-Compulsive Disorder (OCD)

Specific phobias, such as fear of heights or fear of flying, are uncommon in clinical practice and, in our opinion, are best referred to a behavioral therapist. On the other hand, there is evidence that OCD, a particularly dysfunctional condition characterized by compulsive preoccupations with fixed thoughts and with rituals designed to modify anxiety, can be effectively treated with a variety of medications, especially serotonin-specific agonists, such as clomipramine,[14] sertraline,[15] fluvoxamine,[16] and fluoxetine.[17]

In controlled studies, cognitive-behavioral techniques have also consistently been shown to be effective for OCD.[18,19] Behavioral strategies, including exposure to feared situations and thoughts, prevention of rituals, and cognitive-behavior therapy (CBT), are within the expertise of primary care practitioners with appropriate training or may be provided by referral to a collaborating behavioral psychotherapist. In recent studies the two treatments showing the best response in treating OCD are pharmacotherapy with serotonin reuptake inhibitors and CBT using exposure and response prevention.[20] The combination of CBT and medication appears to potentiate treatment efficacy, but it may be more clinically beneficial to introduce CBT after a period of medication than to start both therapies simultaneously.[21] Earlier meta-analytical reviews of treatments for OCD had shown no consistent differences in effectiveness for CBT, medications, or their combination.[22,23]

Social Phobias

In our society, social phobia or social anxiety disorder—a persistent and disproportionate fear in a performance or social setting—is a relatively common psychiatric illness that causes persistent functional impairment and disability in patients who have this disorder.[24,25] The duration of this condition is frequently lifelong, and it has a high degree of co-morbidity with other psychiatric disorders, such as alcoholism.[26] Patients are best treated aggressively with antidepressants that can be tolerated over the long term.[26] These psychopharmacological agents, combined with cognitive-behavioral therapy designed to meet the particular psychological needs of an individual patient, hold significant promise for good clinical results.[27] It is interesting to note that beta blockers have been successfully used for the treatment of symptoms associated with a specific type of social anxiety: performance anxiety.[28]

Posttraumatic Stress Disorder (PTSD)

The essential feature of PTSD is the development of symptoms following exposure to an extremely traumatic stressor that results in intense fear, helplessness, or horror through direct experience, witnessing, or knowledge of an event that involved actual or perceived threat to life or physical integrity.[13] The characteristic symptoms consist of three clusters: persistent reexperiencing of the traumatic event (at least one symptom); avoidance of stimuli associated with the trauma, with numbing of emotions (at least three symptoms); and increased arousal (at least two symptoms).[13]

As much as 90% of the general population are exposed to a traumatic event during their lifetime.[29] Such events include being involved in a life-threatening accident, fire, flood, or natural disaster; serving in combat; being raped, robbed, or physically attacked; and witnessing the death or injury of another person.[30,31] Approximately 20% of women and 8% of men exposed to such events will develop symptoms of posttraumatic stress disorder (PTSD).[31] The estimated lifetime prevalence of PTSD is 10% in women and 5% in men, meaning that one out of every ten women and one out of every twenty men may be affected at some time.[31]

Studies suggest that PTSD is underrecognized in both general medicine and psychiatric clinical practice.[32,33] A recent study found that even subthreshold symptoms of PTSD were associated with increased impairment and co-morbidity and that patients were significantly at risk for suicidal ideation.[34] Many clinicians may identify and treat symptoms of anxiety or depression but may not recognize PTSD when specific symptoms of PTSD are not the presenting complaint.[33] Patients with PTSD are likely to present in a medical office, seeking help for musculoskeletal, gastrointestinal, cardiovascular, pelvic, or neurological complaints.[32] A smaller percentage of patients presents with symptoms of depression, anxiety, or stress.[32] Patients who have undergone untoward medical procedures, such as traumatic birth, a stay in an intensive care unit, or intubation, or have awakened during surgery because of insufficient anesthesia are also at risk of developing PTSD. Other people at high risk for PTSD are those who have learned about or witnessed the sudden or unexpected death of a loved one.

Clinicians should consider PTSD when patients present with somatic symptoms and screen for any history of deeply frightening experiences or physical, sexual, or emotional abuse, as well as for symptoms of depression, other anxiety disorders, and substance abuse disorders.[32] Psychological treatments for PTSD include exposure therapy, cognitive therapy, and anxiety management, which can be undertaken by the primary care practitioner alone or in collaboration with a mental health specialist. Pharmacotherapy has also been somewhat effective, with selective serotonin reuptake inhibitors (SSRIs) holding the most promise. Of these, sertraline (Zoloft) has been approved for use in PTSD.[35]

We would like to emphasize that, as we stated in Chapter 5, early intervention in acute stress disorder has been shown to prevent PTSD.[36] Having a high index of suspicion for PTSD and an understanding of its pathogenesis in acute traumatic situations may, in fact, be the best preventive medicine that can be practiced.

Panic Attack and Panic Disorder

According to DSM-IV, a panic attack is a discrete period of intense apprehension, fear, or terror with at least four of the following thirteen associated symptoms: palpitations or tachycardia; sweating; trembling or shaking; shortness of breath or smothering sensation; choking; chest pain or discomfort; nausea or abdominal distress; dizziness, unsteadiness, lightheadedness, or faintness; depersonalization or derealization; fear of going crazy or doing something uncontrollable; fear of dying; numbness or tingling sensation; and flushes or chills.[13]

Panic attacks usually are of sudden onset and build to a peak rapidly, usually within five to fifteen minutes (although on occasion they can last for hours). These attacks are often accompanied by a sense of imminent danger or impending doom, and afflicted patients have an almost overwhelming urge to escape this situation. Panic attacks, however, are not necessarily diagnostic of panic disorder. The diagnosis of panic disorder can only be confirmed when a patient presents with at least one month of anticipatory anxiety following a single panic attack, worry, or behavioral changes consequent to anxiety attacks. (These symptoms cannot be due to substance abuse or a medical condition.) Panic disorder tends to be a chronic disease that responds to therapy but is also associated with a high rate of relapse over many years. Both psychotherapy and pharmacology are used to treat these patients. Cognitive-behavioral therapy appears to be more effective than other psychological approaches.

Three groups of drugs have proved effective in controlling panic disorder: benzodiazepines, tricyclic antidepressants, and selective serotonin reuptake inhibitors (SSRIs).[5] We recommend that the benzodiazepines be reserved for treating occasional, infrequent panic attacks. Patients find it reassuring to have an effective medication available to them for their immediate use in such a situation. For this purpose we would recommend alprazolam (Xanax) because its high potency and short duration of action make it the benzodiazepine of choice for patients who have to cope with infrequent panic attacks. For many years tricyclic antidepressants have been known to be effective in control of panic disorder, but their side effect profile is such that they are not as commonly used today. Imipramine (Tofranil) appears to be the most studied of these agents, but other tricyclics have been used with comparable results.[37] At the present time the SSRIs are the choice for the long-term treatment of panic disorder. Both sertraline (Zoloft) and paroxetine (Paxil) have indications for panic disorder and are effective, although other SSRIs have been used with some success also. Because of the high relapse rate, long-term pharmacotherapy with the SSRIs, in conjunction with psychotherapy, is the most reasonable way to manage these patients. Long-term therapy is measured in months to years. More than 50% of panic patients receiving medication will need therapy indefinitely, whereas treatment with cognitive-behavioral therapy has been shown to result in remission.[38]

Most anxiety disorders commonly seen in primary care are amenable to combinations of pharmacotherapy and psychotherapy. The choice of agent or technique is at the option of the therapist, but skilled primary care practitioners are reporting good results with judicious use of drug therapy in combination with psychotherapy. A reasonable way to approach patients with anxiety symptoms, from a psychopharmacological perspective, appears at the top of p. 143.[39]

DEPRESSIVE DISORDERS

"As many as 5–10% of primary care patients suffer from major depression at any one time, and another 10–15% will be experiencing lesser degrees of depression."[40] If answers

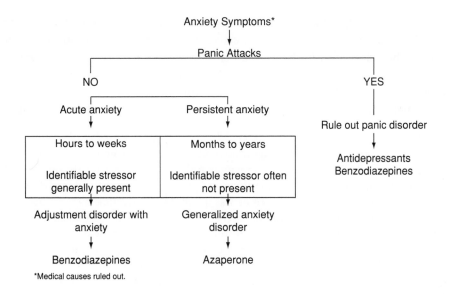

Anxiety Symptoms*
↓
Panic Attacks

NO / YES

NO → Acute anxiety / Persistent anxiety

YES → Rule out panic disorder → Antidepressants / Benzodiazepines

Hours to weeks	Months to years
Identifiable stressor generally present	Identifiable stressor often not present

Acute anxiety → Adjustment disorder with anxiety → Benzodiazepines

Persistent anxiety → Generalized anxiety disorder → Azaperone

*Medical causes ruled out.

to the *BATHE* questions lead the clinician to suspect depression, the popular mnemonic "SIG E CAPS" (for depressed patients the prescription is energy capsules) can be used to confirm the diagnosis[41]:

S	Increased or decreased sleep and decreased **sexual** desire
I	Decreased **interest** or pleasure in almost all activities
G	Inappropriate **guilt** or feelings of worthlessness/hopelessness
E	Decreased **energy** or fatigue
C	Decreased **concentration**
A	Increased or decreased **appetite** with weight gain or loss
P	**Psychomotor** agitation or retardation
S	**Suicidal** ideation, plan, or attempt

If patients have at least five positive symptoms as well as depressed mood or anhedonia, this meets the criteria for a major depression. Many patients seen in primary care will have less severe forms of the disorder. These conditions are known as subthreshold, subsyndromal, mild, or moderate depression or dysthymia (chronic depression "lite"). These can often be treated by cognitive interventions and prescribing regular exercise daily of at least 25 minutes' duration, although adding a suitable antidepressant is always an option.

Since depression is usually accompanied by anxiety, it is fortunate that the agents used to treat depression frequently also have anxiolytic properties. Choosing an agent that has activating or sedating side effects would depend on the patient's presentation. for example, the commonly used antidepressant trazodone (Desyrel) is generally more sedating than the SSRI paroxetine (Paxil), which is more activating. The primary care practitioner needs to know that a number of very good antidepressant agents are available and that all of them have about the same success rate of approximately 70%.[42] The major difference among classes of antidepressants is in the area of side effects. The newer SSRIs and like agents are probably no more effective than many of the products they are replacing, but their side-effect profiles are much better and therefore adherence with treatment regimens is more likely.[43] Likewise, augmentation of one medication with a medication from the same or another class is commonly employed in the treatment of depression with or without concomitant anxiety, since single-drug therapy is not always effective.[44,45]

J.H. is a 42-year-old CPA (certified public accountant) who was seen in the office by a family practice resident for a routine insurance examination. Although he appeared to be quite healthy, he had answered positively to a number of questions on the insurance form relating to symptoms and minor problems related to his health. When he was questioned about these answers, his responses were rather vague and unfocused and did not seem to indicate any particular organ system and/or specified organ dysfunction. His past medical history was unremarkable: he had never been hospitalized, took no medications, and had last seen a physician for a driver's examination when he moved to the state approximately 10 years previously. Because the patient was being seen for an insurance examination, it was awkward for the resident to explore some of these issues.

However, when the resident used the *BATHE* sequence, the patient's answers strongly indicated that he was unhappy and quite probably clinically depressed. The *SIG E CAPS* questions revealed that the patient was indeed "blue," with early-morning awakening, worsening anhedonia, and guilt feelings about his lack of energy. The patient added that he had considerable difficulty getting his day's work done, his memory was "failing him," his appetite was getting consistently worse, and he was getting more nervous and jittery, which further impaired his ability to concentrate. He related that "I just can't keep my mind on anything and I just pace about the office trying to focus but can't do it with any efficiency." When he was directly questioned about whether he had considered harming himself in any way, he responded "no," explaining that he was too afraid of it to think about doing that (although he could understand why people who were suffering like he was would entertain such thoughts).

At this point, the resident strongly advised the patient to see his personal physician because this condition, a clinical depression, was treatable and would only get worse if ignored. The patient responded by asking the resident to be his doctor since he was the first person who had expressed personal interest, seemed to understand the nature of the problem, and appeared to care about how the patient felt. Since the patient had no regular source of care, and once the insurance matter was taken care of there was no conflict of interest, the resident assumed responsibility for the patient's care and initiated treatment.

The treatment regimen consisted of seeing the patient on a regular basis to provide psychological support and the use of both low doses of a benzodiazepine (to handle the patient's immediate problem of jitteriness and jumpiness) and an SSRI (for his underlying depression). Over the next six weeks the benzodiazepines were tapered as the SSRI dose was slightly increased with the patient responding to this approach. Currently the patient is doing well. Because this was the patient's first major depressive episode, medication will be continued for six months to one year, and then it will be tapered and the patient's clinical course monitored. At present the patient is scheduled for regular visits, the resident is making cognitive-behavioral interventions, and both parties are pleased with the positive outcome.

Premenstrual Dysphoric Disorder

Approximately 3% to 5% of menstruating women experience premenstrual dysphoric disorder (PMDD), a disorder with severe premenstrual symptoms that cause significant impairment in social or occupational functioning. This disorder, a subset of premenstrual syndrome (PMS) that occurs in 20% to 50% of menstruating women, is recognized in the DSM-IV as a depressive disorder.[13] PMDD differs from PMS in its requisite mood symptoms, their severity, and their resulting impairment.[13] Obviously, the timing of the symptoms distinguishes PMDD from other depressive disorders, in which symptoms persist throughout the menstrual cycle.[13] For some women, the symptoms generally cause some distress but may not interfere greatly with their lives. These women have mild symptoms and make lifestyle changes in their diet, exercise, and stress management to help control their symptoms. Others have severe symptoms that usually do not respond to conservative interventions.[46]

The diagnosis of PMDD requires a 12-month history of severe discomfort, such as fatigue, sleep and appetite changes, physical symptoms (e.g., breast tenderness, bloating), or difficulty concentrating, as well as an affective symptom (anxiety, depression, irritability, or mood swings) during the luteal phase of the menstrual cycle.[13] These symptoms should disappear soon after menstruation begins, and few to no symptoms should occur during the follicular phase.[13]

Currently, selective serotonin reuptake inhibitors (SSRIs) are the first-line treatment choice for PMDD. Preliminary studies show intermittent administration of clomipramine, fluoxetine, citalopram, or sertraline during the luteal phase of the menstrual cycle is effective in the treatment of PMDD.[47-50] Double-blind, placebo-controlled studies have shown fluoxetine, sertraline, and paroxetine to be effective for full-cycle treatment of PMDD.[51-53] Fluoxetine, currently marketed as Sarafem, is the first SSRI approved by the U.S. Food and Drug Administration (FDA) for the treatment of PMDD.

SUMMING UP THE ANTIDEPRESSANT MEDICATIONS

Because a large number of agents are commonly used in the treatment of depression, (with or without anxiety), Tables 9–1 and 9–2 should be helpful in determining appropriate doses and expected side-effect profiles among various available pharmacological choices.[54]

OTHER CONDITIONS AMENABLE TO PSYCHOPHARMACOTHERAPY

Although the anxiety and depressive disorders constitute the bulk of the mental health problems treated by primary care practitioners, psychotropic medication is useful in treating a number of other conditions. We would like to briefly discuss the role of pharmacotherapy in the treatment of attention-deficit/hyperactivity disorder, Alzheimer's disease, bulimia nervosa, and chronic pain.

Table 9–1 Antidepressant Forms and Dosages

Drug	Dosage Forms (mg)	Initial Dose (mg/day)*	Range (mg/day)	Frequency	Half-Life	Safe in Overdose
Selective Serotonin Reuptake Inhibitors (SSRIs)						
Fluoxetine (Prozac)	10, 20 mg Pulvules, 20 mg/ 5 ml liquid	20	20–60	qd (AM)	2–9 days	Yes
Sertraline (Zoloft)	50, 100 scored tablets	50	50–200	qd	1–4 days	Yes
Paroxetine (Paxil)	10, 20, 30, 40 coated tablets	20	20–50	qd	10–24 hr	Yes
Fluvoxamine (Luvox)	50, 100 scored tablets	50	50–300	qd (hs)	15 hr	Yes
Citalopram (Celexa)	20, 40 scored tablets	20	20–60	qd	35 hr	Yes
Miscellaneous						
Venlafaxine (Effexor)	25, 37.5, 50, 75, 100 scored tablets 37/5, 75, 150 XR (extended release)	75 37.5	75–375 75–375	bid qd (hs)	5–11 hr 5–11 hr	Yes Yes
Nefazodone (Serzone)	100, 150, 200, 250 scored tablets	200	200–600	bid	2–4 hr	Yes
Trazodone (Desyrel)	50, 100, 150, 300 scored tablets	150	150–600	qd (hs)	4–9 hr	Yes
Bupropion (Wellbutrin)	75, 100 tablets 100, 150 SR (sustained release) tablets	200 150	200–450 200–450	tid† bid	8–24 hr 8–24 hr	Yes Yes
Tricyclics						
Amitriptyline (Elavil)	10, 25, 50, 75, 100, 150 coated tablets	50–75	50–300	qd (hs)	31–46 hr	No
Clomipramine (Anafranil)	25, 50, 75 tablets	25	25–250	qd (hs)	19–37 hr	No
Doxepin (Sinequan)	10, 25, 50, 75, 100, 150 capsules, 10 mg/ml solution	50–75	25–300	qd (hs)	8–24 hr	No

		Starting dose*	Dose range	Schedule	Half-life	
Imipramine (Tofranil)	10, 25, 50 coated tablets	50–75	30–300	qd (hs)	11–25 hr	No
Trimipramine (Surmontil)	25, 50, 100 capsules	50–75	50–300	qd (hs)	7–30 hr	No
Desipramine (Norpramin)	10, 25, 50, 75, 100, 150 coated tablets	50–75	25–300	qd (hs)	12–24 hr	No
Nortriptyline (Pamelor)	10, 25, 50, 75 capsules, 10 mg/5 ml solution	25–50	30–100	qd‡	18–44 hr	No
Protriptyline (Vivactil)	5, 10 coated tablets	10–15	15–60	tid	67–89 hr	No
Amoxapine (Asendin)	25, 50, 100, 150 scored tablets	100–150	50–600	qd‡	8 hr	Yes
Tetracyclics						
Maprotiline (Ludiomil)	25, 50, 75 scored tablets	50–75	50–225	qd (hs)	21–25 hr	No
Mirtazapine (Remeron)	15, 30 scored tablets	15	15–60	qd (hs)	20–40 hr	Yes (?)
Monoamine Oxidase Inhibitors						
Phenelzine (Nardil)	15 coated tablets	45	45–90	tid	2–4 hr	No
Tranylcypromine (Parnate)	10 coated tablets	30	30–60	tid	2.4–2.8 hr	No

*Initial daily adult dose. Elderly persons should receive half the starting dose.

†Initial dose 100 mg bid for 3 days, then 100 mg tid.

‡Start in divided doses (tid)—maintenance may be once daily at bedtime (qd [hs]).

Table 9-2 Antidepressant Side Effects

Drug	Antichol-inergia	Sedation	Insomnia/Agitation	Orthostatic Hypotension	Arrhythmia	Nausea	Weight Gain	Sexual Dysfunction
Amitriptyline (Elavil)	++++	++++	0	++++	+++	0	++++	++
Desipramine (Norpramin)	+	+	+	++	++	0	+	+
Doxepin (Sinequan)	+++	++++	0	++	++	0	+++	++
Imipramine (Tofranil)	+++	+++	+	++++	+++	+	+++	++
Nortriptyline (Pamelor)	+	+	0	++	++	0	+	+
Protriptyline (Vivactil)	++	+	+	++	++	0	0	++
Trimipramine (Surmontil)	+	++++	0	++	++	0	+++	+
Amoxapine (Asendin)	++	++	++	++	+++	0	+	++
Maprotiline (Ludiomil)	++	++	0	+	+	0	++	0
Mirtazapine (Remeron)	+	++	0	+	0	0	+++	0
Trazodone (Desyrel)	0	++++	0	+	+	+	+	0
Nefazodone (Serzone)	0	+++	0	+	+	+	0	0
Bupropion (Wellbutrin)	0	0	++	0	+	+	0	0
Venlafaxine (Effexor)	0	0	++	0	0	++	0	+
Fluoxetine (Prozac)	0	0	+++	0	0	+++	0	++
Paroxetine (Paxil)	0	0	+++	0	0	+++	0	++
Sertraline (Zoloft)	0	0	+++	0	0	+++	0	++
Fluvoxamine (Luvox)	0	0	+++	+	0	+++	0	++

Modified from Depression Guideline Panel. *Depression in Primary Care: Detection, Diagnosis, and Treatment: Quick Reference Guide for Clinicians.* No. 5. U.S. Department of Health and Human Services publication no. 93-0552. Rockville, Md.: Agency for Health Care Policy and Research, 1993.
0, None; +, minimal; ++, mild; +++, moderate; ++++, strong.
*Over 13 lb.

Attention-Deficit/Hyperactivity Disorder

There is considerable controversy, particularly in the lay literature, about the use of stimulants for attention-deficit/hyperactivity disorder (ADHD), a neurobehavioral syndrome characterized by developmentally inappropriate degrees of inattentiveness, impulsivity, and hyperactivity.[55] At the present time, the exact cause of ADHD is unknown, but considerable research is under way because of the relatively common occurrence of this disorder and its impact on the patient, family, and community at large. This disorder may affect as many as 10% of school-based youths.[56] A recent analysis conducted by the Council on Scientific Affairs of the American Medical Association concluded that, overall, there is "little evidence of widespread overdiagnosis or misdiagnosis of ADHD or of widespread overprescription of methylphenidate by physicians."[57] The American Academy of Pediatrics contends that use of stimulants is indicated when the child's or adolescent's behavior is impairing that individual's ability to learn and/or develop interpersonal relationships. However, the academy cautions that drug therapy should not be used alone, but rather it needs to be integrated as part of a comprehensive approach to the patient (including proper classroom placement, behavior modification, and counseling).[58]

Methylphenidate (Ritalin) is the stimulant most commonly associated with the pharmacological treatment of ADHD, but a variety of other agents, including pemoline (Cylert), dextroamphetamine (Dexedrine Spansule), extended-release methylphenidate (Concerta), and amphetamine mix (Adderall), are also used and with reported effectiveness. A recent study indicates that there would be much less controversy about medication for ADHD if clinicians were consistently implementing both medication and evidence-based behavioral interventions.[59] Since nontreatment of affected individuals has the potential for catastrophic outcomes, we recommend judicious use of stimulants along with close follow-up and support as the treatment of choice.

Alzheimer's Disease

Dementia of the Alzheimer's type (DAT), characterized by progressive multiple cognitive deficits, is the most commonly occurring dementia, accounting for approximately 50% of patients evaluated for progressive cognitive decline.[40] The impact of Alzheimer's disease on patients, families, and communities can be devastating. From its insidious onset, manifested by increasingly frequent memory loss and impaired judgment, the disease is unrelenting, eventually robbing patients of their personality and families of their quality of life.

The judicious use of pharmacotherapy for cognitive dysfunction and behavioral disturbances in Alzheimer's disease can be of some help but should also be accompanied by strong efforts to provide education and support for the patient, the family, and other caregivers.[60] The psychopharmacological agents include two acetylcholinesterase inhibitors, tacrine (Cognex) and donepezil (Aricept), as well as ergoloid mesylates (Hydergine) and a variety of over-the-counter ginkgo biloba products. These products have no really profound impact on the progression of Alzheimer's disease but have been shown to provide some relief, and consideration should be given to their use.[60,61]

Bulimia Nervosa

The essential features of bulimia nervosa are binge eating and inappropriate compensatory methods to prevent weight gain.[13] This is a disease of the middle and upper classes and primarily affects young women. Although bulimia is not as pervasive as the tabloids would have one believe, primary care practitioners will encounter an occasional patient with this disorder. Since individuals with bulimia nervosa are typically ashamed of their eating problems and attempt to conceal their symptoms,[13] the practitioner must have a high index of suspicion for this disorder and ask patients specific questions about their eating habits and body image.

The approaches to treatment of bulimia nervosa are cognitive-behavioral, pharmacological, and a combination of the two.[62] At present, cognitive-behavioral therapy is recognized as the most effective treatment for bulimia nervosa.[63] A practitioner who feels comfortable with and is trained in this area can provide the treatment or refer to a mental health specialist. However, regardless of the type of therapist, the use of antidepressants should also be considered as an adjunct to psychotherapy. Combination treatment of antidepressants and psychotherapy has been associated with significantly greater improvement in binge frequency and depressive symptoms than either treatment alone.[64]

Managing Chronic Pain

Patients complaining of chronic pain and seeking drugs to ameliorate their suffering can present quite an unwelcome challenge to the primary care practitioner. Much has been made lately of the issue of pain. Media attention has been focused on the topic with implications that the medical profession is not paying enough attention to this area of patient care. Perhaps this is the legacy of an earlier age when influences on medical practice saw pain as good: an opportunity to purge the soul. It is currently recognized that pain detracts from the quality of life and that it can, and should, be treated. The Joint Commission on Accreditation of Healthcare Organizations (JCAHO) has gone so far as to revise their standards to ensure that "pain is assessed in all patients."[65] Many consider pain to be the "fifth vital sign."

When thinking of pain most clinicians think of acute pain and the use of analgesics, antiinflammatory agents (including NSAIDs), and narcotics, either alone or in combination, to relieve patients' suffering. In the treatment of chronic pain and pain-producing conditions such as fibromyalgia it is particularly important to avoid the use of addicting drugs. Along with cognitive-behavioral treatments, success has been reported in using the antidepressant amitriptyline (Elavil), 25 mg to be taken two to three hours before bedtime.[66] Although the exact relationship among tricyclic antidepressants, neurotransmitters, and pain is not thoroughly understood, the reality is that these medications are effective in many cases and worthy of consideration.

ANSWERING PATIENTS' QUESTIONS CONCERNING PSYCHOTROPIC HERBS*

Herbal medicines, or phytotherapeutics, are often used by patients to treat depression and any related symptoms. It is important to ask patients about use of herbals and neutraceuticals and to be nonjudgmental when eliciting this information, since patients often do not share this information with their practitioners. A "don't ask, don't tell" attitude can produce adverse outcomes, since phytotherapeutics exhibit distinct pharmacological effects.

St. John's wort (*Hypericum perforatum*) is used for symptoms of depression and dysthymia.[67] It appears to be effective in the treatment of mild to moderate depression but not for severe depression.[68] It induces the cytochrome P-450 3A4 enzyme system, so drug interactions with other medications using the same enzyme system have to be considered in patients taking St. John's wort. Most reported side effects are of a serotonergic nature, so patients need to be warned not to combine prescribed antidepressants with St. John's wort.[69]

SAMe (S-adenosyl-methionine) is used for depression, osteoarthritis, and other chronic pain syndromes. Its effectiveness for the treatment of depression has not yet been well established, and interactions can occur with prescription antidepressants.[70,71]

Kava (*Piper methysticum*) is used to treat anxiety disorders, insomnia, and musculoskeletal pain syndromes. It seems to be effective for these indications, but long-term use (more than one month) without physician supervision should be avoided.[72] Valerian root is used for mild anxiety and insomnia. It seems to be effective for these indications; it is characterized by a slow onset of action, often over a period of six weeks, much like SSRIs.[67,73]

Unfortunately, herbal products vary widely in quality, purity, and price. Until regulatory agencies and the botanical industry responsibly address these issues, patients will experience variable outcomes not necessarily related to the efficacy of the particular herb. Patients should be advised to look for standardized products when appropriate, as well as a certificate of analysis. The parts of the herb used should be specified and the contents in milligrams listed on the bottle. If patients are frail or elderly, the dosages of herbals might need to be reduced, much like pharmacological agents.[69]

SUMMARY

Although a variety of psychopharmacological agents are effective for treating mental health problems, optimal patient care requires that they be used along with psychological support, talk, and other behavioral interventions. Where feasible, pharmacotherapy is most useful for getting patients through the acute phase of a disorder. The DSM-IV of the American Psychiatric Association lists a number of disorders that could be reasonably managed by a primary care clinician who employs both pharmacotherapy and "talk therapy." These conditions include anxiety, depression, attention-deficit/hyperactivity disorder, bulimia, and Alzheimer's disease. Although anxiety and depression are traditionally

---

*We wish to express our sincere appreciation to Beatrix Roemheld-Hamm, M.D., Ph.D., for her assistance with this section.

classified as distinct entities, they are frequently found in combination and should be treated with a psychopharmacological agent that is effective for both conditions. The SWIKIR Anxiety Scale is proposed as a relatively quick and efficient method for the primary care clinician to use to identify a patient suffering from anxiety when the *BATHE* sequence uncovers a problem. Included in the anxiety disorders that can be effectively managed in primary care are adjustment disorder with anxiety, generalized anxiety disorder, social phobia, posttraumatic stress disorder, and panic disorder. The *SIG E CAPS* mnemonic is a tool for helping to establish the diagnosis of depression in patients when the *BATHE* sequence indicates that this may be the patient's problem. Major depressive disorders; subthreshold, subsyndromal, minor depression or dysthymia; and premenstrual dysphoric disorder are all depressive disorders that can be effectively managed by the primary care clinician, with or without a collaborating mental health professional. In addition to the anxiety and depressive disorders, primary care clinicians can be expected to treat (again, either alone or in collaboration with a mental health specialist) obsessive-compulsive disorder, attention-deficit/hyperactivity disorder, Alzheimer's disease, bulimia nervosa, and chronic pain. It is important to determine if patients are self-medicating with herbal products.

References

1. Pincus, H.A., Tanielian, T., Marcus, S., Olfson, M., Zarin, D.A., Thompson, J., & Magno Zito, J. Prescribing trends in psychotropic medications: Primary care, psychiatry and other medical specialties. *Journal of the American Medical Association*, 1998, *279*(7), 526–531.
2. Keller, M.B., McCullough, J.P., Klein, D.N., Arnow, B., Dunner, D., Gelenberg, A., Markowitz, J.C., Nemeroff, C.B., Russell, J.M., Thase, M.E., Trevedi, M.H., & Zajecka, J. A comparison of nefazodone, the cognitive behavioral-analysis system of psychotherapy, and their combination for the treatment of chronic depression. *New England Journal of Medicine*, 2000, *342*(20), 1462–1470.
3. Kessler, R.C., McGonagle, K.J., Zhao, S., Nelson, C.B., Hughes, M., Eshleman, S., Wittchen, H.U., & Kendler, K.S. Lifetime and 12-month prevalence of DSM-III-R psychiatric disorders in the United States. *Archives of General Psychiatry*, 1994, *51*, 8–19.
4. Greenberg, P.E., Sisitsky, T., Kessler, R.C., Finkelstein, S.N., Berndt, E.R., Davidson, J.R.T., Ballenger, J.C., & Fyer, A.J. The economic burden of anxiety disorders in the 1990's. *Journal of Clinical Psychiatry*, 1999, *60*(4), 427–435.
5. Feighner, J.P. Overview of antidepressants currently used to treat anxiety disorders. *Journal of Clinical Psychiatry*, 1999, *60*(suppl. 22), 18–22.
6. McRae, A.L., & Brady, K.T. Review of sertraline and its clinical applications in psychiatric disorders. *Expert Opinion Pharmacotherapy*, 2001, *2*(5), 883–892.
7. Gorman, J.M., & Papp, L.A. Efficacy of venlafaxine in mixed depression-anxiety states. *Depression Anxiety*, 2000, *12*(suppl. 1), 77–80.
8. Baughman, O.L. Rapid diagnosis and treatment of anxiety and depression in primary care: The somatizing patient. *Journal of Family Practice*, 1994, *39*(4), 373–378.
9. Schweizer, E., & Rickels, K. Strategies for treatment of generalized anxiety in the primary care setting. *Journal of Clinical Psychiatry*, 1997, *58*(suppl. 3), 27–31.
10. Uhlenhuth, E.H., Balter, M.B., Ban, T.A., & Yang, K. International study of expert judgment on therapeutic use of benzodiazepines and other abuse liability of benzodiazepines in the long-term treatment of anxiety disorders. *Journal of Clinical Psychopharmacology*, 1999, *19*(6, suppl. 2), 23S–29S.
11. Goisman, R.M. Psychosocial treatment prescriptions for generalized anxiety disorder, panic disorder, and social phobia, 1991–1996. *American Journal of Psychiatry*, 1999, *156*, 1819–1821.

12. Ewing, J.A. Detecting alcoholism: The CAGE questionnaire. *Journal of the American Medical Association*, 1984, *252*(14), 1905–1907.

13. *Diagnostic and Statistical Manual of Mental Disorders*, 4th ed. (DSM-IV). Washington, D.C.: American Psychiatric Association, 1994.

14. Clomipramine Collaborative Study Group. Clomipramine in the treatment of patients with obsessive-compulsive disorder. *Archives of General Psychiatry*, 1991, *48*, 730–738.

15. Chouinard, G., Goodman, W., Greist, J., Jenike, M., Rasmussen, S., White, K., Hackett, E., Gaffney, M., & Bick, P.A. Results of a double-blind placebo controlled trial of a new serotonin uptake inhibitor, sertraline, in the treatment of obsessive-compulsive disorder. *Psychopharmacology Bulletin*, 1990, *26*, 279–284.

16. Perse, T.L., Greist, J.H., Jefferson, J.W., Rosenfeld, R., & Dar, R. Fluvoxamine treatment of obsessive-compulsive disorder. *American Journal of Psychiatry*, 1987, *144*, 1543–1548.

17. Tollefson, G.D., Rampey, A.H., Potvin, J.H., Jenike, M.A., Rush, A.J., Dominguez, R.A., Koran, L.M., Shear, M.K., Goodman, W., & Genduso, L.A. A multicenter investigation of fixed-dose fluoxetine in the treatment of obsessive-compulsive disorder. *Archives of General Psychiatry*, 1994, *51*, 559–567.

18. Fals-Stewart, W., Marks, A.P., & Schafer, J. A comparison of behavioral group therapy and individual behavior therapy in treating obsessive-compulsive disorder. *Journal of Nervous and Mental Disease*, 1993, *181*, 189–193.

19. Van Oppen, P., de Haan, E., Van Balkom, A.J.L.M., Spinhoven, P., Hoogduin, K., & van Dyck, R. Cognitive therapy and exposure in vivo in the treatment of obsessive compulsive disorder. *Behavior Research and Therapy*, 1995, *33*(4), 379–390.

20. Mathew, S.J., Simpson, H.B., & Fallon, B.A. Treatment strategies for obsessive-compulsive disorder. *Psychiatric Annals*, 2000, *30*(11), 699–708.

21. O'Connor, K., Todorov, C., Robillard, S., Borgeat, F., & Brault, M. Cognitive-behaviour therapy and medication in the treatment of obsessive-compulsive disorder. *Canadian Journal of Psychiatry*, 1999, *44*(1), 564–571.

22. Cox, B.J., Swinson, R.P., Morrison, B., & Lee, P.S. Clomipramine, fluoxetine, and behavior therapy in the treatment of obsessive-compulsive disorder: A meta-analysis. *Journal of Behavioral Therapy and Experimental Psychiatry*, 1993, *24*, 149–153.

23. van Balkom, A.J., van Oppen, P., Vermeulen, A.W., & van Dyck, R. A meta-analysis on the treatment of obsessive-compulsive disorder: A comparison of antidepressants, behavior, and cognitive therapy. *Clinical Psychology Review*, 1994, *14*, 359–381.

24. Keck, P., & McElroy, S. New uses for antidepressants: Social phobia. *Journal of Clinical Psychiatry*, 1997, *58*(suppl. 14), 32–36.

25. Tancer, M., & Uhde, T. Role of serotonin drugs in the treatment of social phobia. *Journal of Clinical Psychiatry*, 1997, *58*(suppl. 5), 50–54.

26. Pollack, M.H. Comorbidity, neurobiology, and pharmacotherapy of social anxiety disorder. *Journal of Clinical Psychiatry*, 2001, *62*, 24–29.

27. Juster, H., & Heinberg, R. Social phobia. *Psychiatric Clinics of North America*, 1995, *18*(4), 821–840.

28. Jefferson, J.W. Social phobia: A pharmacologic treatment overview. *Journal of Clinical Psychiatry*, 1995, *56*(suppl. 5),18–24.

29. Breslau, N., Kessler, R.C., Chilcoat, H.D., Schultz, L.R., Davis, G.C., & Andreski, P. Trauma and posttraumatic stress disorder in the community: The 1996 Detroit Area Survey of Trauma. *Archives of General Psychiatry*, 1998, *55*(7), 626–632.

30. Solomon, S.D., & Davidson, J.R.T. Trauma: Prevalence, impairment, service use and cost. *Journal of Clinical Psychiatry*, 1997, *58*(suppl. 9), 5–11.

31. Kessler, R.C., Sonnega, A., Bromet, E., Hughes, M., & Nelson, C.B. Posttraumatic stress disorder in the National Comorbidity Survey. *Archives of General Psychiatry*, 1995, *52*, 1048–1060.

32. Samson, A.Y., Bensen, S., Beck, A., Price, D., & Nimmer, C. Posttraumatic stress disorder in primary care. *Journal of Family Practice*, 1999, *48*(3), 222–227.

33. Zimmerman, M., & Mattia, J.I. Is post-traumatic stress disorder underdiagnosed in routine clinical settings? *Journal of Nervous and Mental Diseases*, 1999, *187*, 420–428.

34. Marshall, R.D., Olfson, M., Hellman, F., Blanco, C., Guardino, M., & Struening, E.L. Comorbidity, impairment and suicidality in subthreshold PTSD. *American Journal of Psychiatry*, 2001, *158*(9), 1467–1473.

35. Brady, K., Pearlstein, T., Asnis, G.M., Baker, D., Rothbaum, B., Sikes, C.R., & Farfel, G.M. Efficacy and safety of sertraline treatment of posttraumatic stress disorder: A randomized controlled trial. *Journal of the American Medical Association*, 2000, *283*(14), 1837–1844.

36. Bryant, R.A., Sackville, T., Dang, S., Moulds, M., & Guthrie, R. Treating acute stress disorder: An evaluation of cognitive behavior therapy and supportive counseling techniques. *American Journal of Psychiatry*, 1999, *156*(11), 1780–1786.

37. Barlow, D.H., Gorman, J.M., Shear, M.K., & Woods, S.W. Cognitive-behavioral therapy, imipramine, or their combination for panic disorder: A randomized controlled trial. *Journal of the American Medical Association*, 2000, *283*, 2529–2536.

38. Marks, I.M., Swinson, R.P., Basoglu, M., Kuch, K., Noshirvani, H., O'Sullivan, G., Lelliott, P.T., Kirby, M., McNamee, G., Sengun, S., & Wickwire, K. Alprazolam and exposure alone and combined in panic disorder with agoraphobia: A controlled study in London and Toronto. *British Journal of Psychiatry*, 1993, *162*, 776–787.

39. Hales, R.E., Hilty, D.A., & Wise, M.G. A treatment algorithm for the management of anxiety in primary care practice. *Journal of Clinical Psychiatry*, 1997, *58*(suppl. 3), 76–80.

40. Goldman, L.S., Wise, T.N., & Brody, D.S. *Psychiatry for Primary Care Physicians*. Chicago: American Medical Association, 1998, p.77.

41. Wise, M.G., & Rundell, J.R. *Concise Guide to Consultation Psychiatry*, 2nd ed. Washington, D.C.: American Psychiatric Press, 1994, pp. 55–56.

42. Hales, R.E., Yudofsky, S.C., & Talbott, J.A. *The American Psychiatric Press: Textbook of Psychiatry*, 3rd ed. Washington, D.C.: American Psychiatric Press, 1999, p. 1029.

43. Goldman, L.S., Wise, T.N., & Brody, D.S. *Psychiatry for Primary Care Physicians*. Chicago: American Medical Association, 1998, p. 339.

44. Yudofsky, S., Hales, R.E., & Ferguson, T. *What You Need to Know About Psychiatric Drugs*. Washington, D.C.: American Psychiatric Press, 1991, p. 53.

45. Fava, M. Augmentation and combination strategies in the treatment of refractory depression. *Journal of Clinical Psychiatry*, 2001, *62*, 4–11.

46. Korzekwa, M.I., & Steiner, M. Premenstrual syndromes. *Clinical Obstetrics and Gynecology*, 1997, *40*, 564–576.

47. Steiner, M., Korzekwa, M., Lamont, J., & Wilkins, A. Intermittent fluoxetine dosing in the treatment of women with premenstrual dysphoria. *Psychopharmacology Bulletin*, 1997, *33*, 771–774.

48. Wikander, I., Sundblad, C., Andersch, B., Dagnell, I., Zylberstein, D., Bengtsson, F., & Eriksson, E. Citalopram in premenstrual dysphoria: Is intermittent treatment during luteal phases more effective than continuous medication throughout the menstrual cycle? *Journal of Clinical Psychopharmacology*, 1998, *18*(5), 390–398.

49. Young, S.A., Hurt, P.H., Benedek, D.M., & Howard, R.S. Treatment of premenstrual dysphoric disorder with sertraline during the luteal phase: A randomized, double-blind, placebo-controlled crossover trial. *Journal of Clinical Psychiatry*, 1998, *59*(2), 76–80.

50. Jermain, D.M., Preece, C.K., Sykes, R.L., Kuehl, T.J., & Sulak, P.J. Luteal phase sertraline treatment for premenstrual dysphoric disorder. *Archives of Family Medicine*, 1999, *8*(4), 328–332.

51. Freeman, E.W., Rickels, K., Arrendondo, F., Kao, L-C., Pollack, S.E., & Sondheimer, S.J. Full or half cycle treatment of severe premenstrual syndrome with a serotonergic antidepressant. *Journal of Clinical Psychopharmacology*, 1999, *19*(1), 3–8.

52. Pearlstein, T.B., Stone, A.B., Lund, S.A., Scheft, H., Slotnick, C., & Brown, W.A. Comparison of fluoxetine, bupropion, and placebo in the treatment of premenstrual dysphoric disorder. *Journal of Clinical Psychopharmacology*, 1997, *17*(4), 261–266.

53. Freeman, E.W., Rickels, K., Sondheimer, S.J., & Polansky, M. Differential response to antidepressants in women with premenstrual syndrome/premenstrual dysphoric disorder. *Archives of General Psychiatry*, 1999, *56*, 932–939.

54. Rakel, R.E. Depression. *Primary Care Clinics in Office Practice, Mental Health*, 1999, *26*(2), 219–220.

55. Adesman, A.R. The diagnosis and management of attention-deficit/hyperactivity disorder in pediatric patients: Primary care companion. *Journal of Clinical Psychiatry*, 2001, *3*(2), 66–77.

56. Wolraich, M.L., Hannah, J.N., Pinnock, T.Y., Baumgaertel, A., & Brown, J. Comparison of diagnostic criteria for attention-deficit hyperactivity disorder in a county-wide sample. *Journal of the American Academy of Child and Adolescent Psychiatry*, 1996, *35*(3), 319–324.

57. Goldman, L.S., Genel, M., Bezman, R.J., & Slanetz, P.J. Diagnosis and treatment of attention-deficit/hyperactivity disorder in children and adolescents. *Journal of the American Medical Association*, 1998, *279*(14), 1100–1107.

58. American Academy of Pediatrics Committee on Children with Disabilities, Committee on Drugs. Medication for children with attention disorders. *Pediatrics*, 1996, *98*, 301–304.

59. Evans, S.W., Pelham, W.E., Gnagy, E.M., Smith, B.H., Bukstein, O., Greiner, A.R., Altenderfer, L., & Baron-Myak, C. Dose-response effects of methylphenidate on ecologically valid measures of academic performance and classroom behavior in adolescents with ADHD. *Experimental and Clinical Psychopharmacology*, 2001, *9*(2), 163–175.

60. Rakel, R.E. *Conn's Current Therapy 2000*. Philadelphia: Saunders, 2000, p. 844.

61. Le Bars, P.L., Katz, M.M., Berman, N., Itil, T.M., Freedman, A.M., & Schatzberg, A.F. A placebo-controlled, double-blind, randomized trial of an extract of *Ginkgo biloba* for dementia: North American EGb Study Group. *Journal of the American Medical Association*, 1997, *278*(16), 1327–1332.

62. Mcgilley, B.M., & Pryor, T.L. Assessment and treatment of bulimia nervosa. *American Family Physician*, 1998, *57*(11), 2743–2750.

63. Agras, W.S., Crow, S.J., Halmi, K.A., Mitchell, J.E., Wilson, G.T., & Kraemer, H.C. Outcome predictors for the cognitive behavior treatment of bulimia nervosa: Data from a multisite study. *American Journal of Psychiatry*, 2000, *157*(8), 1302–1308.

64. Bacaltchuk, J., Trefiglio, R.P., Oliveira, I.R., Hay, P., Lima, M.S., & Mari, J.J. Combination of antidepressants and psychological treatments for bulimia nervosa: A systematic review. *Acta Psychiatrica Scandinavica*, 2000, *101*(4), 256–264.

65. Joint Commission on Accreditation of Healthcare Organizations. *2001 Comprehensive Accreditation Manual for Hospitals*. Oakbrook Terrace, Ill.: The Commission, 2001, p. PE-8.

66. Godfrey, R.G. A guide to the understanding and use of tricyclic antidepressants in the overall management of fibromyalgia and other chronic pain syndromes. *Archives of Internal Medicine*, 1996, *156*, 1047–1052.

67. Blumenthal, M., Busse, W.R., Goldberg, A., Gruenwald, J., Hall, T., Riggins, C.W., & Rister, R.S. *The Complete German Commission E Monographs: Therapeutic Guide to Herbal Medicines*. Boston: American Botanical Council, 1998.

68. Shelton, R.C., Keller, M.B., Gelenberg, A., Dunner, D.L., Hirschfeld, R., Thase, M.E., Russell, J., Lydiard, R.B., Crits-Cristoph, P., Gallop, R., Todd, L., Hellerstein, D., Goodnick, P., Keitner, G., Stahl, S.M., & Halbreich, U. Effectiveness of St. John's wort in major depression: A randomized controlled trial. *Journal of the American Medical Association*, 2001, *285*(15), 1978–1986.

69. Schulz, V.R., & Hansel, V.E. *Rational Phytotherapy: A Physician's Guide to Herbal Medicine*, 3rd ed. Berlin: Springer, 1998.

70. Iruela, L.M., Minguez, L., Merino, J., & Monedero, G. Toxic interaction of S-adenosylmethionine and clomipramine. *American Journal of Psychiatry*, 1993, *150*(3), 522.

71. Jellin, J.M., Gregory, P., Batz, F., Hitchens, K., Burson, S., Shaver, K., & Palacioz, K. *Pharmacist's Letter/Prescriber's Letter Natural Medicines Comprehensive Database*, 3rd ed. Stockton, Calif.: Therapeutic Research Faculty, 2000

72. Brinker, F. *Herb Contraindications and Drug Interactions*, 2nd ed. Sandy, Ore.: Eclectic Medical Publications, 1998.

73. Donath, F., Quispe, S., Diefenbach, K., Maurer, A., Fietze, I., & Roots, I. Critical evaluation of the effect of valerian extract on sleep structure and sleep quality. *Pharmacopsychiatry*, 2000, *33*(2), 47–53.

CHAPTER 10

Therapeutic Interventions for Difficult Patient Situations

Now that we have discussed pharmacological interventions, it is time to focus on some of the more difficult patient encounters. There are patients who are hard to treat because they are hard to be with. There are hostile patients, addicted patients, anxious and depressed patients who may or may not take medication, chronic pain patients, and suicidal patients who pose a danger to themselves, to mention only a few. How can we relate to them? And what do we do with those patients suffering from the current "disease of the month," whether chronic fatigue, fibromyalgia, or another somatization disorder? Can we really do anything for them? What is more important, can we help them without feeling put upon—without feeling depleted and less able to relate with genuine empathy to other patients?

Also, what, if anything, can we do to treat children and adolescents reacting to the circumstances of their lives? First, how do we get them to talk? Then, what do we do with the information?

A word of caution is in order. The techniques outlined in this chapter build on previous material. The practitioner must have acquired a thorough understanding and reasonable comfort level using our supportive techniques in routine patient care before applying these specific approaches to the care of their most difficult patients. Providing supportive psychotherapy is a skill that needs to be practiced consistently and applied broadly to all patients.

REACTING TO DIFFICULT PATIENTS

Over 20 years ago Groves[1] wrote an article provocatively titled "Taking Care of the Hateful Patient," in which he developed four stereotypes of particularly difficult patient personalities and behavioral categories. The four stereotypes are dependent clingers, manipulative help-rejecters, entitled demanders, and self-destructive deniers. Such individuals precipitate negative feelings on the part of practitioners, who feel depleted by the need to provide endless emotional supplies without achieving any objective positive outcome. After grouping differences and similarities, Groves developed specific approaches for dealing with each of these patient types. Our approach is much simpler. We start with the notion that each patient is behaving in the best possible way, for this patient, at this time and will make fundamental changes only when properly motivated either in response to catastrophe or by a series of small steps. We will try to create an environment to precipitate the small steps.

Keeping Sessions Brief

Except in situations posing an immediate threat to life or limb, we suggest that practitioners limit contact with patients who arouse negative emotions to no more than 10 or 15 minutes, regardless of the complexity of the problems or lists of complaints. During that time the practitioner is encouraged to integrate medical and psychosocial concerns, treating the patient in the context of the total life situation. If there are too many problems for one visit, the patient can be brought back the following week. This strategy has the additional advantage of demonstrating the practitioner's interest. It addresses the patient's needs in a supportive manner. Patients will feel less rejected (and these patients are highly skilled at getting clinicians and others to reject them) if they are provided with frequent brief sessions. Ultimately this will result in much better utilization of time, since there will not be lengthy and frustrating sessions of miscommunication. Ultimately patients will learn to organize the details of their stories to fit into the time available. Practitioners may have to take charge quite directly by saying something such as "I can hear that you have several things that really bother you. You have some abdominal pains that come and go. You feel all shaky inside and are upset that there is so little cooperation at home. That sounds like a lot for you to deal with. However, I need to understand what, specifically, you would like me to do for you today."

Approaching the Situation Differently

Reframing problem situations as opportunities for growth and skill development is a healthy stress management technique we have been promoting in this book. So, rather than thinking, "Oh, good grief, Mrs. Brown is on my schedule. I hate to see her since she has numerous problems, doesn't take her medicine, never feels grateful, never gets better or stops complaining," we can think, "Oh, it's Mrs. Brown. I feel sorry that she is so needy. Seeing her will give me an opportunity to try out some of these new techniques I'm learning. I will let her talk about two minutes. I will paraphrase what she has said so she will know I listened. Then, after I find out what is going on in her life and acknowledge her suffering, I will ask her to concentrate on one specific problem and try to get her to identify one small change that she can make to make herself feel better. If I can make the time with her more productive, I will feel good. I will aim for one small win and limit the time with her to no more than 15 minutes."

When practitioners learn to reframe situations and take satisfaction from dealing with difficult patients in a smooth and effective manner, the practice of medicine may well become gratifying again. Seeing people relax and become less anxious, hostile, or demanding is a tremendous experience. As we change our approach, unreasonable patients often become more reasonable.

Understanding the Patient's Emotional Context

Patients are sometimes unpleasant, critical, and hostile. For some, this is a personality style. Many times, however, patients are frustrated because they are not feeling or functioning well or because they experience chronic symptoms. They may be unhappy with limits set by their insurance carriers or hassles involved in obtaining care. They may also be tired of being dependent on care providers who are not always able to help them. In response, they become hostile. They are so sure that they will not get their needs met that their attitude and behavior ensure completion of this self-fulfilling prophecy. It is important to note that an appropriate empathic intervention will break this pattern. Acknowledging the patient's frustration instead of demanding that it be held in check immediately changes the situation. Let us look at some practical examples.

THE HYPOCHONDRIACAL PATIENT

Perhaps the most difficult patients to deal with, over time, are the hypochondriacal patients, whose preoccupation with real or imagined illness tries the patience of the most dedicated practitioner.[2,3] A.J. Barsky and his colleagues found that hypochondriacal patients are dissatisfied with their physicians, that physicians are frustrated by the patients, and that the use of the term "hypochondriasis" impairs "the physician's accuracy in assessing the levels of the patient's anxiety and depression."[4] Hypochondriacs suffer from anxiety and depression particularly because they exaggerate their appraisal of disease risk, jeopardy, and vulnerability.[3] They define good health as a condition of being entirely symptom-free and consider any symptoms, no matter how transitory, as indicative of sickness.[5] These patients focus much of their time and attention on monitoring their physical symptoms and suffer acutely while being unsuccessful in finding anyone to cure them. Hypochondriacs need to be scheduled for regular visits at predetermined intervals (for starters, every two weeks is often tolerable for both patient and practitioner) whether or not they are experiencing disturbing symptoms. Over time the interval between visits can be increased.

Informing these patients that they will receive regular care whether or not they are feeling acutely ill is the first positive step in managing hypochondriasis. Regular sessions preempt the patient's need to develop new symptoms with which to engage the practitioner. After acknowledging patients' concerns about their current symptoms and emphasizing that it must be awful to never feel well, the practitioner must follow the *BATHE* protocol during every visit.

These patients may become defensive and insist that the stress in their lives is not what is causing their symptoms. The practitioner should not argue about this. On the contrary, it is important to agree with the patient but to express concern that given how badly the patient feels it must be difficult to cope with everything that is going on and that stress has a major effect on all illness. Once elicited, psychosocial data should be recorded so that inquiries can be made about outcomes of situations in the patient's life. This communicates that the practitioner is interested in the patient as a person and not just as a collection of disease symptoms. The patient does not have to be sick to get attention or a response. As the relationship progresses, the practitioner may wish to explore the patient's unrealistic expectations regarding his or her state of "health."[5]

As we have said, it is important to acknowledge patients' physical suffering and to allow them a reasonable amount of time to discuss it, to prescribe symptom relief, but always to put things back into the context of the patient's life: "How does that affect your ability to spend time with your grandchildren?" "What can you do to maximize enjoyment during the times when you feel reasonably good?" "What might you do to distract your mind and give you at least some temporary relief from your worry?"

Over time, this approach may offer these patients the opportunity to focus on other aspects of life besides physical complaints. Their previous life experience may have led these patients to believe that care and attention could only be gotten through illness-related behavior. Now there are alternatives. By structuring visits regularly and including broader aspects of the patient's experience, the practitioner can treat the hypochondriac quite successfully. We again caution practitioners not to let the length of the session exceed their own tolerance for contact with this type of patient. Perhaps it will be necessary to limit the time to seven or eight minutes. The session would start with the practitioner making this clear: "Mrs. Brown, we have about eight minutes. Tell me what you are most concerned about this week." Since there are regularly scheduled visits, each session can focus on one or two problems. Our experience has been that patients respond very well to this type of treatment. After a while, they will tolerate longer periods between visits but will usually need to be seen at least once every six weeks, or they will regress. It is also important to allow these patients to keep at least one or two symptoms. P. Watzlawick[6] has pointed-ed out how critical it is to always allow patients the unresolved remnant.

THE CHRONIC COMPLAINER

There is a subtle difference between hypochondriacs who are truly anxious regarding the state of their health (sometimes referred to as the "worried well") and chronic complainers,[7] troublesome patients who have multiple complaints, feel the need to be seen frequently, and fit into the category of entitled demanders, so aptly described by Groves.[1] These patients rarely get well and never seem to appreciate the efforts that the practitioner makes on their behalf. It would appear obvious that these patients need their disease in order to function at all, as seen by the following example:

Mary S. has been seeing Dr. L. for almost eight months on a regular basis. She is a 47-year-old, divorced, obese, white female, with moderately well-controlled hypertension, who also complains of insomnia and a variety of aches and pains. Mary had been laid off from her job as a factory worker and been put on temporary disability payments. She is very angry because her benefits are about to expire and she has problems paying her rent, argues constantly with her 21-year-old son who lives with her, and feels that her married daughter and son-in-law treat her badly. Mary talks loudly and fast. It is as though she wants to get 20 minutes of conversation into a 10-minute session. Dr. L. usually feels as though he has been assaulted, or perhaps run over by a lawn mower, after spending any amount of time with her.

Routine lab work and careful examination have convinced Dr. L. that Mary's problems are primarily stress-induced, stress that she generates for herself and others. He has developed a clinical style that allows his patient the first minutes of the interview to complain about whatever is bothering her most, after which he takes control and examines one problem in detail. After monitoring medications and "laying on hands," in the process of a brief physical examination, Dr. L. wonders what Mary could do differently in a specific interaction with her son. He sees her regularly, every two weeks. Her improvement is obvious, and she is starting to become aware that she has power to make things happen, and not just by being demanding. There are even indications that since she feels accepted she is learning to listen (a little).

There is a growing body of contemporary literature focusing on somatization disorders.[8-14] The basics of psychosomatic medicine were first proposed in a 1943 article by Franz Alexander in which he explained that some patients experiencing internal conflicts but not free to express certain emotions, such as anger, fear, frustration, neediness, or sorrow, developed the physical symptoms that were concomitants of the emotion.[15] Psychiatrists contend that once these emotions can be expressed directly, the need to somatize will decrease.[16] Studies evaluating utilization of outpatient medical services have consistently documented high utilization by patients who somatize and experience psychological distress as physical.[17-20]

We know that the stress response (and the stress can be self-induced, as it is with the chronic complainer) will activate physiological reactions that both are acutely felt and can become chronic and ultimately precipitate organic problems. Patients experience physiological symptoms that result from sympathetic arousal that does not get discharged productively. Many patients do not know how to get any kind of care or attention without complaining. Sadly, when their complaints are not effective, they persevere and complain louder and longer, further increasing their stress.

Life stress has been shown to be predictive of increased medical care utilization for all patients, but particularly for somatizers.[21] J. Miranda and colleagues have suggested that outpatient medical services need to focus on teaching stress reduction as a way to manage this problem. The effectiveness of cognitive stress management interventions that help people to reinterpret situations, thereby changing the actual emotional reaction, becomes obvious. Until patients become aware of the mechanisms involved and the power to ameliorate their reactions, they are trapped. Anyone who is trapped or pushed into a corner is not very nice to deal with. Therapeutic interventions by practitioners that empower patients and slowly, over time, convince them that they can affect their health, emotions, and the course of their lives, and directly get their needs met other than by complaining about symptoms are extremely effective.

When the chronic complainer bemoans the fact that his wife offers him no sympathy, the practitioner can respond, "I can see that that is very difficult for you. What is it, specifically, that you want from your wife?"

Patient: "I want her to pay attention to me."
Practitioner: "That makes sense. Does she pay attention when you tell her about your pain?"
Patient: "No, she ignores me. Then she starts complaining about her headaches."
Practitioner: "I see. Can you think of something you could do to change the situation?"

If the patient responds negatively, it is important not to argue. Power struggles are not useful. When we convince patients that they are wrong, we lose, because we damage the patients' self-esteem. In Chapter 3, we pointed out the enormous power that is attributed to practitioners. This power that can be used therapeutically to great advantage can also be used detrimentally, to diminish the patient.

It is best to try to get the patient to commit to doing one small task that has a positive and realistic potential. When the patient says that his wife complains about her headaches, perhaps the patient could give her the kind of sympathetic response that he desires. It would certainly get her *attention*.

One of the great challenges of outpatient medicine is that practitioners have no control over what patients do after they leave the office. If patients are not committed, they will sabotage the practitioner's best efforts. Practitioners must convince patients about the importance of changing a behavior, that change is possible, and that there is a payoff for trying. Assignments must be broken down into modest, feasible tasks, and then small wins will accumulate, reinforce the patient's efforts, and make big differences.

BEHAVIORAL TREATMENT FOR ANXIETY

According to the late Gabe Smilkstein, M.D., "Anxiety is the enemy of health."[22] Anxiety is a signal that the body sends to warn of danger. The signal is real and its manifestations are scary, but the danger is often nonexistent or self-induced. Nevertheless, this fear signal results in somatic arousal. It is the discomfort with and further fear of arousal that make this a clinical problem. When patients experience somatic arousal, they tend to engage in behavioral avoidance of situations that precipitate these sensations. They also assume certain cognitions (catastrophic beliefs) that have been linked to depression and symptom severity in somatizing patients.[23] These behavioral and thought patterns result in a lack of self-efficacy, anticipatory inadequacy, and hypervigilance.

Many effective treatments for anxiety exist, both pharmacological and behavioral. It is imperative to assure the patient that the varied symptoms are all real and frightening but can be managed. As discussed in Chapter 9, medication effectively treats the symptoms of somatic arousal, leading to improved functioning. However, when patients learn to control their symptoms through relaxation training and cognitive restructuring, meditation, establishing hierarchies of feared situations, or engaging in regular exercise programs, their levels of arousal will be diminished.[24] Patients can be taught diaphragmatic breathing and progressive muscle relaxation and be asked to practice these techniques for 15 minutes twice daily. The practitioner can also encourage patients to become aware of their thoughts, to monitor those thoughts for distortions (generalizing, "awfulizing," and "catastrophizing"), and to substitute more positive or functional thoughts. Once the patient becomes aware that the negative and frightening ideas, not the actual situation, are precipitating their anxiety, the practitioner can teach the patient to challenge these thoughts by reflecting on one or more of the following questions from the work of Beck and Emery[25]: (1) What is the evidence? (2) What is another way to look at the situation?

(3) All right, what if that does happen? This is another area where *bibliotherapy*,[26] such as reading books from Appendix B, can be very helpful. When patients acquire psychological insight into their condition and learn techniques that make them feel that they can control their symptoms, they will feel safer. There will be less need to pay constant attention to avoid danger. Sometimes it will be necessary for patients to make major life changes in order to escape from situations that are truly destructive. Having the practitioner as a sounding board can be very supportive.

For symptomatic relief while the patient is learning skills or preparing to make life changes to reduce the source of the anxiety Beck and Emery[25] suggest using the A-W-A-R-E technique to help patients label and accept their anxiety. The elements of A-W-A-R-E are as follows:

A. Accept the anxiety.
W. Watch your anxiety. Rate the anxiety on a scale from 0 to 10, and watch it change.
A. Act with the anxiety. Act as if you are not anxious. Breathe normally and slowly.
R. Repeat the steps until the anxiety goes down to a comfortable level.
E. Expect the best.

Having a structure for dealing with the symptoms of somatic arousal puts the patient back in control. This is also a useful strategy for practitioners to use personally when dealing with anxious patients.

Stress Management 101

We would like to be absolutely clear as to what is involved in the practice of stress management. The first prerequisite for managing stress is to become aware that one is experiencing tension. This can be done by gently scanning areas of the body where tension is usually felt—for example, the back between the shoulder blades, neck, temples, or lower back. Overt symptoms indicating stress generally involve rapid and shallow breathing, muscle tension, and racing thoughts. Therefore stress management consists of deliberately taking slow, deep breaths, relaxing the muscles, and modifying the thought process. Breathing techniques and progressive muscle relaxation are easily learned techniques that simply require brief daily practice over a period of perhaps two weeks. Racing thoughts are managed with cognitive-behavioral strategies. These techniques require patients to modify their perceptions and interpretations of various situations; in other words, to change their stories. Patients learn to monitor their thought patterns and to recognize when their thinking is unduly negative. They can then challenge their unrealistic assumptions (horror stories) and substitute more realistic, appropriate, and adaptive versions.

TREATING THE SUBSTANCE-ABUSING PATIENT

Substance abuse continues to be a major problem in U.S. society although the "drug of choice" may vary over time.[27] Treating the alcohol or narcotics abuser is difficult because, by definition, these patients do not exercise control or take responsibility for their behavior. Four questions useful in helping to make a diagnosis of alcoholism focus on asking about *Cutting down, Annoyance by criticism, Guilt feelings,* and *Eye-openers.* The acronym "CAGE" helps the practitioner to recall the questions.[28] The questions can be modified to detect problems with other types of chemicals. When screening elicits evidence of a serious problem, the practitioner may wish to refer the patient to an appropriate treatment program.

If a practitioner wishes to personally manage the treatment for this type of patient, the patient must accept responsibility for attempting to run away from, rather than dealing with, pain or problematic situations in his or her life. Recognizing that this has created an additional problem rather than a solution is the first step in the patient's recovery. Next, the patient must agree to accept help and to diligently follow the instructions of the practitioner. Substance abusers are not generally capable of mustering the resources to solve problems by themselves. The first constructive step in overcoming a substance abuse problem is for the patient to admit helplessness to control the addiction and to accept help from an outside source.[29] A firm contract must be made with the patient committing to abstinence from the drug of choice (or other nonprescribed chemicals), following the practitioner's orders explicitly, and agreeing to honestly report any infringement of these conditions. Firm limits must be set, and the contract depends on the patient's compliance. The patient's involvement in a 12-step support group will increase the odds of success dramatically.

Helping Patients to Change Their Behavior

Whether patients are abusing alcohol or tobacco, maintaining a sedentary lifestyle, eating the wrong foods, or engaging in other destructive health habits, practitioners must be mindful of the fact that people will not change their behavior until they are ready to do so. This means that the individual has to see the necessity or benefit, consider it possible, and feel it is safe to do so (it will not result in a loss of "face"). Clearly, using power tactics is futile. We recommend two strategies.

First, if a behavior is destructive, the practitioner should inquire at every visit whether the patient has "thought about" changing the particular behavior. If the patient says "yes," this can be reinforced with "Good. That's the first step. You might think about when you might want to actually do it." If the patient says, "I've tried and I can't," the response must be "You just haven't been successful *yet.*" Use of the word "yet" will help patients attain the "contemplative stage," which is a prerequisite for changing behavior.[30]

The second strategy involves giving patients a homework assignment to construct a decision balance.[31] This means listing all the benefits and risks of the current behavior and the perceived benefits and risks (losses of pleasure, friends, etc.) of the changed behavior. These can then be discussed at the next visit. Until patients recognize that the benefits of changing their behavior clearly outweigh the effort involved, no lasting, positive outcome can be expected.

THE DEPRESSED PATIENT

Having to spend time with depressed patients can be very depressing. It is even more depressing to read that long-term follow-up studies show that depression *not* diagnosed or treated by primary care practitioners is highly associated with long-lasting symptomatology, decreased quality of life, and suicide.[32] Not all depressions are major ones, but even mild to moderate depressions negatively affect people's lives. Depression can be treated very effectively using brief sessions. Since there is something contagious in the negativity, heaviness, hopelessness, and neediness expressed by these unhappy people, it is important to set realistic expectations for both patient and practitioner. The patient can be expected to suffer but can be encouraged to make some small changes, minute ones if necessary. D.C. Klein and M.E.P. Seligman[33] demonstrated conclusively that getting people to successfully accomplish small tasks can reverse the learned helplessness (the story based on past experience that there is nothing to be done to escape a bad situation) that is the correlate of depression.

Thus, in treating a depressed patient, we first give the patient permission to be depressed. We do *not* suggest that these patients should feel any differently than they do. If they could, they would. We do *not* focus these patients on the positive features of their lives. That only sets up resistance and guilt. We do *not* point out that other people also have horrible problems. Depressed people do not care about the experience of others. We *do* tell the family to stop trying to cheer the patient up. Patients who are depressed and are told to look on the bright side of things, or to count their blessings, often feel misunderstood, wrong, ungrateful, unworthy, or any number of unpleasant feelings, which exacerbates their depression. Instead, we agree that it seems as though *right now* things are really bad and state that we can understand that the patient would feel awful. Sometimes, if we are lucky, the patient will actually respond with something positive. Perversity is an endemic human quality.

Certainly, if necessary, the practitioner can prescribe an antidepressant as described in Chapter 9. However, while waiting for the medication to take effect and subsequently along with the medical treatment, behavioral suggestions and cognitive therapy will be very effective. Behavioral treatment might start by suggesting one activity that will give the patient a subjective sense of control: "I want you to get some exercise, take a brisk walk, perhaps 10 minutes, twice daily. It is not required that you enjoy it, you just have to do it." "Do one small thing for yourself each day." "Make a list of all the tasks you have to do and feel that you can't. Then do just one. The one that takes the least time." "Forget about mornings, you probably will feel rotten, but plan to do one constructive thing every afternoon." If there has been a previous history of depressive episodes, it is useful to ask, "What sort of things did you do previously that helped you to feel better?"

Cognitive therapy consists of challenging some of the negative assumptions and generalities that the patient makes. The practitioner will agree that right now things look very bad but there is no evidence to show that they will always be that way. Focus on the fact that the patient has an illness and that the illness will resolve. Whenever the patient makes a negative statement, the practitioner can edit the statement by inserting the word "yet." "Yes, I understand that you have not been able to motivate yourself to exercise, yet." "No, your appetite has not improved, yet." The implication that things will change—that the patient is not stuck in the internal, stable, global explanatory box—is very powerful. The practitioner's confidence stirs hope in the patient. Anxiety may be the enemy of health, but *hope is the antidote for depression.*

Depressed patients often believe that the world has to be a certain way before they will be able to function adequately, and they become immobilized in the meantime. Cognitive interventions focus on defining the specific problem, devising one or more solutions, and in the meantime helping patients achieve a more functional state of coping with whatever is going on. A homework assignment might specify that the patient walk at least 30 minutes daily, do something pleasurable no less than once each week, and read the first three chapters of David Burns's *Feeling Good*[34] (see Appendix B).

The practitioner must not expect to change the patient's situation but must contract to see the patient regularly, be supportive (lead to the patient's strength), prescribe and monitor medications (if appropriate), and set reasonable limits on the patient's allowable worrying and wallowing time. Labeling worrying and wallowing for what they are and setting a five-minute limit on these types of activity at any given time are very effective.

THE GRIEVING PATIENT

In Chapter 6 we pointed out that grief work can usually be accomplished in six to eight sessions. Whenever a patient appears to be overreacting to a current loss, an unresolved grief reaction or possibly a posttraumatic stress disorder (see Chapter 9) may be contributing to the severity of the response. The practitioner needs to probe in order to ascertain if this is true. If so, it is important to explain to the patient the significance of completing the mourning process and how difficult this can sometimes be.

Grief work can be very difficult for the patient. First, it is painful. Moreover, although all people feel some ambivalence toward the significant others in their lives, most people are uncomfortable with the anger that is generated when they experience abandonment through death or other circumstances. Conversely, when a troubled relationship ends in divorce or separation, patients may be uncomfortable when they experience a sense of loss and longing for the positive aspects. It is important that patients talk about these feelings and that they review the significant aspects of the lost relationship.

The six or eight sessions do not necessarily have to occur weekly. In a resistant patient, either because of reluctance to experience the intense pain or because the patient is in denial about the significance of the loss, the practitioner can simply bring up the subject briefly every time the patient is seen for any medical problem. However, ideally, the patient will be cooperative and willing to work. Because grief work does requires a thorough airing of the issues and reminiscing about important details, homework in the form of writing about the person or the details of the loss can be very helpful.[35] Talking to relatives or friends, reviewing snapshots, and visiting significant places can be very beneficial. The 15-minute session with the practitioner is then used to highlight important understandings.

The patient is doing the work on his or her own time and simply recording the progress with the practitioner. As stated previously, the grieving process involves reviewing the significant aspects of the loss, coming to terms with both the good and bad aspects of what is gone, feeling the pain, accepting the finality of the event, and finally letting go.

Anniversary reactions are extremely common, and patients benefit from being warned to expect a variety of somatic symptoms and mood shifts around the anniversary date of a loss or other significant event.[36] Effective treatment simply involves encouraging patients to feel and accept their pain, rather than trying to shut it off. It is helpful to explain that pain comes in waves, will pass, and does diminish over time and to state explicitly, "You will not always feel this way." Basically, all that is required of both the patient and the practitioner is just to be there.

THE SUICIDAL PATIENT

When working with depressed or grieving patients, we must consider suicide a potential risk, but we will never know if they are suicidal if we do not ask. These patients are experiencing such high levels of subjective pain that the desire to turn off this pain may make the option of killing themselves appear to be quite attractive. In general, serious consideration of suicide corresponds with serious feelings of poor self-esteem, lack of social support, and lack of hope. People who talk about suicide will do it, if their attempts to get help fail.

In our experience primary care practitioners can treat potentially suicidal patients very effectively. Once these patients feel that someone is really concerned about them, they readjust their notions that there is no one in the world who cares and that everyone would be better off if they were dead. The practitioner acknowledges that suicide is always an option, that it may seem desirable at a given time, but that once exercised, suicide excludes all other options. Since it is always better to keep one's options open, the practitioner might say, "I hate to see you use a permanent solution for what may turn out to be a temporary problem. Let's keep your options open. Why don't we see how you feel in a few weeks? Let's take it one day at a time, and see if together, we can find a better way to deal with this situation."

It is imperative to check whether the patient has a plan. If so, the patient must be willing to *commit* to postponing action or will have to be hospitalized for his or her safety. Even with a potential plan, the therapeutic connection with the practitioner can be powerful enough to overcome the feelings of hopelessness and demoralization leading to thoughts of suicide.

The practitioner who chooses to treat a potentially suicidal patient must be available for the patient should the patient need to feel connected. If the clinician is going to be away and someone else will be on call, the covering practitioner must be informed about the seriousness of the situation and the support that must be given. It is hoped that family and friends will also be mobilized. As an assignment, the patient is told to ask for support from significant others. It is important to have the patient verify a commitment to call at a particular time or to come in for an appointment in two days or whatever time period is mutually agreeable. The patient must be given clear instructions to call at a specific time when the practitioner will be personally available to talk.

In general, a patient's promise to call or come in at a specific future time can be safely interpreted as a statement that the patient expects to be around at that time. The patient commits to not harming himself or herself in the interim. A note to that effect must be put into the chart: "Patient promises to call tomorrow to check in. Will be seen on Wednesday for follow-up. Will take no action before further in-person discussion. Patient instructed to go to the emergency room if situation worsens." The patient can be asked to sign the note.

TREATING CHILDREN

When we say that every patient should be *BATHE*d, that includes children. It is often fascinating to compare what a child tells us about what is going on to the story that we get from the adults in the family. Often the discrepancy can be used to make an effective intervention. Asking children what is happening in their lives, how they feel about it, what troubles them the most, and how they are handling it and then giving them empathy establish a wonderful rapport. Sometimes we can help them to interpret the situation differently; other times we can intervene with the parent using the principles outlined in Chapter 8.

Young children or children who are reluctant to talk can be asked to draw a picture. Since children usually draw what is important to them, asking them to tell a story about the picture provides an easy way to get useful information and to connect with the child.[37] Asking a child to draw a person[38] or to draw a family is a lovely way to keep a child occupied while examining a parent and can be used to screen for developmental or situational problems. The practitioner asks the child to "tell me about this family." The practitioner can ask about the various people in the drawing. How do they feel about each other? What makes them happy? What makes them sad? What do they do when they get mad at each other? The practitioner can ask the child, "If you could change one thing, what would it be?" Except in unusual circumstances, interventions focused on changing the parents' behavior toward the child (see Chapter 8) are more efficient and effective than trying to engage the child in a psychotherapeutic relationship. When a case is difficult, referral to a collaborating family therapist is an option to consider.

TREATING ADOLESCENTS AND YOUNG ADULTS

The practitioner should inform parents of young teenagers that it is important to establish a separate relationship with the adolescent. Every visit must include time without the parent in the examining room. Establishing confidential relationships with teenagers is paramount in gaining their trust and respect. Continuity in the relationship also helps. Teenagers can be *BATHE*d around issues of home, school, peers, and their ambitions.

Since the potential for violence in our society is so high, P. Stringham suggests that in addition to routine questions about illness, friends, religion, smoking, alcohol, drugs, gambling, sexual activity, depression, and suicidal thoughts or actions, it is important to ask, "Have you ever been forced to have sex against your will?" and "How many pushing and shoving fights have you had with anyone in the past year?"[39] Screening for violence in relationships and teaching assertive alternatives are important interventions that primary care practitioners can make.

It is important to support adolescents' self-esteem and to acknowledge the difficulty of sorting out the many choices that have to be made on a daily basis. The practitioner can act as a trusted advisor or encourage the adolescent to find another adult (not the parent) to fulfill that role. Teenagers can also be advised to keep journals to record their feelings and experiences. If teenagers are angry with their parents, they must be cautioned not to self-destruct just to get back at their parents. In general, parents should be told to stop nagging (since it does not do any good) and stop criticizing (since it does harm). Teenagers and young adults respond equally well to our techniques. Practitioners in college health services have reported exceptionally good results using our methods, an example of which follows:

Dr. A. assumed that Ken was fairly healthy because this was his first visit to the office since his college health physical and he was now a member of the junior class. His presenting request that "I would like to have my blood pressure checked" was a bit unusual, particularly when, as a matter of routine, the college nurse had checked his vital signs and found them to be textbook "normal." After dispensing with the usual amenities Dr. A. got to the issue of Ken's concern about his blood pressure and quickly ascertained that his problem was fatigue, which he interpreted as a sign of "low blood pressure." Further questioning about the duration and nature of his fatigue, his work and sleep habits, and related symptomatology was less productive except that Dr. A. got the sense that something was disturbing Ken. He struck gold when he used the *BATHE* technique:

Dr. A.: "Ken, what is going on in your life?"

Ken: "Well, Doc, my roommate and his girlfriend are using our room to do their thing; it's gotten to the point that I can't even get in there to get a good night's sleep."

Dr. A.: "How do you feel about that?"

Ken: "It makes me really angry; I am paying for that room, and I can't even use it."

Dr. A.: "What troubles you the most about that?"

Ken: "Well, he claims that he is not keeping me out; both he and his girlfriend suggested that my new girlfriend and I join them but we're just not ready to take that step in our relationship."

Dr. A.: "How are you handling that?"

Ken: "Not well, I mean I am not getting very much sleep, and I'm getting more and more irritated. It's beginning to affect my grades as well as my relationship with my girlfriend."

Dr. A.: "That must be very difficult for you."

When Ken acknowledged that it was, Dr. A. suggested that he think about what other options he could exercise. Ken returned the following week to report that he had a long talk with his roommate and that they had come to an agreement that Ken was comfortable with. Ken was feeling very good about himself and how he handled the situation. Ken thanked Dr. A. for his support. He said that he could not have done it without Dr. A.

Just supporting Ken and making him aware that he had other options empowered him to do what he had to do to solve his own problem, which is generally the case. Chapter 11 will look at how to reconcile the needs of the patient with those of other family members.

SUMMARY

In taking care of difficult patients, awareness that these patients are attempting to solve problems in the best way they can is helpful. Setting limits regarding the length of the visit and the number of problems discussed and reframing the situation as an opportunity for learning help the practitioner cope.

Hypochondriacs suffer from anxiety and depression, particularly because they exaggerate their appraisal of disease risk, jeopardy, and vulnerability. Scheduling them for regular appointments and exploring the context of their lives along with their symptoms are effective treatment. Their suffering is acknowledged, and they are allowed to retain one or two symptoms. Chronic complainers are recognized as needing their disease, but they are encouraged to make small changes that help them feel more in control of their lives.

To successfully treat substance abusers, strict limits must be set. Patients will only modify their behavior when they are ready to do so, but strategies can be employed that will encourage them to contemplate making a change. Overt symptoms indicating stress generally involve rapid and shallow breathing, muscle tension, and racing thoughts. Stress management generally consists of deliberately taking slow, deep breaths, relaxing the muscles, and modifying the thought process. Depressed patients must be given permission to be depressed, while being encouraged to make small changes in the circumstances of their lives. Grieving patients are advised to examine the significant aspects of their terminated relationships and actively mourn their losses. In order to heal, they need to feel their pain, rather than trying to shut it off.

Serious consideration of suicide generally corresponds with feelings of poor self-esteem, lack of social support, and lack of hope. The practitioner counters these by a show of concern and a commitment to help. A contract is made, and the patient promises to call or come in at a specific time. Clear documentation and backup are required.

Children and teenagers can be *BATHE*d during a regular office visit. Children's drawings help to facilitate communication with the practitioner. Although it is essential to respect teenagers' confidentiality, it is also important to screen for interpersonal violence and high-risk behaviors and to support constructive anger management.

REFERENCES

1. Groves, J.E. Taking care of the hateful patient. *New England Journal of Medicine*, 1978, *298*, 883–887.
2. Barsky, A.J., & Klerman, G.L. Overview: Hypochondriasis, bodily complaints, and somatic styles. *American Journal of Psychiatry*, 1983, *140*, 273–283.
3. Barsky, A.J., Ahern, D.K., Bailey, E.D., Saintfort, R., Liu, E.B., & Peekna, H.M. Hypochondriacal patients' appraisal of health and physical risks. *American Journal of Psychiatry*, 2001, *158*, 783–787.

4. Barsky, A.J., Wyshak, G., Latham, K.S., & Klerman, G.L. Hypochondriacal patients, their physicians, and their medical care. *Journal of General Internal Medicine*, 1991, *6*, 413–419.

5. Barsky, A.J., Coeytaux, R.R., Sarnie, M.K., & Cleary, P.D. Hypochondriacal patients' beliefs about good health. *American Journal of Psychiatry*, 1993, *150*, 1085–1089.

6. Watzlawick, P. *The Language of Change: Elements of Therapeutic Communication*. New York: Basic Books, 1978, p. 73.

7. Rittelmeyer, L.F., Jr. Coping with the chronic complainer. *American Family Practitioner*, 1985, *31*, 211–215.

8. Lipkin, M. Functional or organic? A pointless question. *Annals of Internal Medicine*, 1969, *71*, 1013–1017.

9. Cavenar, J.O., Jr., Nash, J.L., & Maltbie, A.A. Anniversary reactions presenting as physical complaints. *Journal of Clinical Psychiatry*, 1978, *39*, 369–374.

10. Barsky, A.J., III. Patients who amplify bodily sensations. *Annals of Internal Medicine*, 1979, *91*, 63–70.

11. Allen, L.A., Gara, M.A., Escobar, J.I., Waitzkin, H., & Silver, R.C. Somatization: A debilitating syndrome in primary care. *Psychosomatics*, 2001, *42*(1), 63–67.

12. Miller, A.R., North, C.S., Clouse, R.E., Wetzel, R.D., Spitznagel, E.L., & Alpers, D.H. The association of irritable bowel syndrome and somatization disorder. *Annals of Clinical Psychiatry*, 2001, *13*(1), 25–30.

13. Crofford, L.J. The hypothalamic-pituitary-adrenal stress axis in fibromyalgia and chronic fatigue syndrome. *Rheumatology*, 1998, *57*(suppl. 2), 67–71.

14. Heim, C., Ehlert, U., Hanker, J.P., & Hellhammer, D.H. Abuse-related posttraumatic stress disorder and alterations of the hypothalamic-pituitary-adrenal axis in women with chronic pelvic pain. *Psychosomatic Medicine*, 1998, *60*, 309–318.

15. Alexander, F. Fundamental concepts of psychosomatic research: Psychogenesis conversion, specificity. *Psychosomatic Medicine*, 1943, *5*, 205–210.

16. Fenichel, O. *The Psychoanalytic Theory of Neurosis*. New York: W.W. Norton & Co., 1945.

17. Fink, P., Sorensen, L., Engberg, M., Holm, M., & Munk-Jorgensen, P. Somatization in primary care: Prevalence, health care utilization, and general practitioner recognition. *Psychosomatics*, 1999, *40*(4), 330–338.

18. Escobar, J.I., Golding, J.M., Hough, R.L., Karno, M., Burnam, M.A., & Wells, K.B. Somatization in the community: Relationship of disability and use of services. *American Journal of Public Health*, 1987, *77*, 837–840.

19. Kroenke, K., Arrington, M.E., & Mangelsdorff, A.D. The prevalence of symptoms in medical outpatients and the adequacy of therapy. *Archives of Internal Medicine*, 1990, *150*, 1685–1689.

20. Labott, S.M., Preisman, R.C., Popovich, J., Jr., & Iannuzzi, M.C. Health care utilization of somatizing patients in a pulmonary subspecialty clinic. *Psychosomatics*, 1995, *36*, 122–128.

21. Miranda, J., Perez-Stable, E.J., Munoz, R.F., Hargreaves, W., & Henke, C.J. Somatization, psychiatric disorder, and stress in utilization of ambulatory medical services. *Health Psychology*, 1991, *10*, 46–51.

22. Smilkstein, G. *Caveat: Patient Centered Care: Theme-Day Presentation*. Society of Teachers of Family Medicine 25th Annual Spring Conference, St. Louis, April 25, 1992.

23. Hassett, A.L., Cone, J.C., Patella, S.J., & Sigal, L.H. The role of catastrophizing in the pain and depression of women with fibromyalgia syndrome. *Arthritis and Rheumatism*, 2000, *43*, 2493–2500.

24. Barlow, D.H. *Anxiety and Its Disorders: The Nature and Treatment of Anxiety and Panic*. New York: Guilford Press, 1988.

25. Beck, A.T., & Emery, G. *Anxiety Disorders and Phobias: A Cognitive Perspective*. New York: Basic Books, 1985.

26. Wright, J., Clum, G.A., Roodman, A., & Febbraro, G.A. A bibliotherapy approach to relapse prevention in individuals with panic attacks. *Journal of Anxiety Disorders*, 2000, *14*(5), 483–499.

27. Johnson, R.A., & Gerstein, D.R. Initiation of use of alcohol, cigarettes, marijuana, cocaine, and other substances in US birth cohorts since 1919. *American Journal of Public Health*, 1998, *88*(1), 27–33.

28. Ewing, J.A. Detecting alcoholism: The CAGE questionnaire. *Journal of the American Medical Association*, 1984, *252*(14), 1905–1907.

29. Brickman, P., Rabinowitz, V.C., Karuza, J., Jr., Coates, D., Cohn, E., & Kidder, L. Models of helping and coping. *American Psychologist*, 1982, *37*, 368–384.

30. Prochaska, J.O., & DiClemente, C.C. Transtheoretical therapy: Toward a more integrative model of change. *Psychotherapy Research Theory & Practice*, 1982, *19*, 276–287.

31. Botelho, R.J., Skinner, H.A., Williams, G.C., & Wilson, D. Patients with alcohol problems in primary care. *Primary Care Clinics in Office Practice, Mental Health*, 1999, *26*(2), 279–298.

32. Murphy, J.M., Olivier, D.C., Sobol, A.M., Monson, R.R., & Leighton, A.H. Diagnosis and outcome: Depression and anxiety in a general population. *Psychological Medicine*, 1986, *16*, 117–126.

33. Klein, D.C., & Seligman, M.E.P. Reversal of performance deficits and perceptual deficits in learned helplessness and depression. *Journal of Abnormal Psychology*, 1976, *85*, 11–26.

34. Burns, D. *Feeling Good*. New York: Morrow, 1980.

35. Pennebaker, J.W., Kiecolt-Glaser, J.K., & Glaser, R. Disclosure of traumas and immune function: Health implications for psychotherapy. *Journal of Consulting and Clinical Psychology*, 1988, *56*, 239–245.

36. Bornstein, P.E., & Clayton, P.J. The anniversary reaction. *Diseases of the Nervous System*, 1972, *33*, 470–472.

37. Gardner, R.A. *Psychotherapeutic Approaches to the Resistant Child*. New York: Jason Aronson, 1975.

38. Mortensen, K.V. *Form and Content in Children's Human Figure Drawings: Development, Sex Differences, and Body Experience*. New York: New York University Press, 1991.

39. Stringham, P. Domestic violence. *Primary Care Clinics in Office Practice, Mental Health*, 1999, *26*(2), 373–384.

CHAPTER 11

Practical Therapeutic Interventions for Special Situations, Staff, and Practitioner

Having looked at ways to manage some of the most difficult patients, it is now time to consider a myriad of collateral problems, such as dealing with family members, especially when they present a self-righteous or divided front. Are there ways to handle these situations smoothly? We think so. They depend largely on following the principles we have discussed earlier. This chapter will focus on constructive approaches that can be taught to nurses, receptionists, and other staff members to cut down on patients' frustration and anxiety. Finally, we will address the application of psychotherapeutic (cognitive) principles as they apply to the practitioner. Managing our own stress and using every problem as an opportunity for personal growth are prerequisites for coaching patients in these skills.

HANDLING DIFFICULT FAMILY MEMBERS

Dealing with the patient's family can be one of the most rewarding or most frustrating aspects of practicing medicine. Often family members will call and provide unsolicited information about a patient or make suggestions about treatment. The confidentiality issue is clear in this situation. Practitioners may not share information about the patient, but they may feel stressed by the lack of clarity regarding their relationship to family members. In general, it is important for practitioners to avoid power struggles and confrontations. Although family members can be assumed to have their own agenda, the practitioner is not responsible for figuring out their issues or making judgments as to their merit.

The Art of Verbal Aikido

Handling family members and avoiding power struggles are important considerations. We recommend that the practitioner learn to practice "verbal aikido." Aikido is a Japanese martial art sometimes referred to as "the dance." When a person who is skilled in aikido is attacked, instead of absorbing a frontal blow, the automatic response is to step to the side and turn quickly, join with the attacker, and follow along in the direction of the attack. Then, after a few seconds, the aikido master gently turns both himself or herself and the attacker around, so that they are both going in the opposite direction. After this, the master can gracefully disengage or knock the attacker out.

Verbally, this translates into always acknowledging the legitimacy of others' requests or positions. It catches them off guard and leaves them open to hearing what the practitioner has to say. By first showing respect for the family member's position and anxiety, the practitioner defuses any potential defensiveness. So, when making treatment or discharge plans or discussing anything with a family member, including the behavior of teenagers, we suggest that the practitioner automatically start with the phrase "I can hear how concerned you are, but . . . (then state your case)." If it is more comfortable, you may prefer to say "I know you care a great deal about your mother (father, husband, son, aunt, niece, grandmother, etc.), but . . . ."

It is irrelevant whether you actually subscribe to the above statement. Making the statement is an effective strategy that gets you the other person's attention and positive receptivity. The same thing can be accomplished by starting with the phrase "I agree with you that . . . (and find some part of their suggestion that you can accept)."

Start by Expressing Agreement

People hear better when someone starts by agreeing with them. The critical issue here is that the more difficult and demanding family members are—regardless of whether you see any merit in their suggestions or even feel that they have a legitimate stake in the outcome—there is nothing to be gained by direct antagonism. Hence this technique is effective.

You may say to yourself, "That drunken bum hasn't given two hoots about his mother in the last five years. Why should he tell me how to treat her?" You may be *absolutely right*, but it will be more difficult to deal with the son if you confront him with that. Instead, you can say, "I can see how concerned you are. This must be very difficult for you. I am really glad you are letting me know what you would like me to do, but my impression (clinical judgment, good medical practice) demands that I do such and such. I will keep you informed." This deprives the other person of ammunition for attacking you. In a later section, "Confronting the Patient," we will discuss the technique for direct confrontation, which should be done only when absolutely necessary. A second verbal aikido technique is to respond to every unacceptable request with the phrase "I *wish* I could do that!" This implies that you are not arbitrarily saying "no," that the request is not unreasonable, and that you care about the well-being of the person doing the asking. It is a very good way of disarming people and avoiding endless arguments. If a family member does continue to insist, it is only necessary to repeat, "I wish I could do that."

Relieving Guilt Is a Therapeutic Intervention

Another important consideration when dealing with families is that often there are large elements of guilt. When the son from Chicago suddenly calls you and demands that absolutely everything be done for his father, whom he has neglected for years, it is a clear sign that an attempt is being made to resolve guilt. We recommend that practitioners absolve family members of guilt whenever possible. Very often it stems from projected resentment. In any case, however, guilt is such an unpleasant emotion that a concomitant hostility is generated toward the person who "makes us" feel guilty. Actually, guilt and hostility are opposite sides of the same coin. It is always therapeutic to say, "I feel confident that you did as much as you could." That is always true. It may not have been enough for the other person, but if the guilty individual could have done more (given his or her story about the relationship), it would have happened. Do not say, "You have no reason to feel guilty." The guilty person is likely to argue. Just say, "I'm sure that you've expressed your love, as best you could. No one can expect more than that."

Enjoying the Challenge

All these interventions are designed to facilitate communications but allow us to practice according to our best judgment. As in aikido, instead of meeting the opponent head-on and absorbing the impact of a direct blow, we come from the side, join in the other's movement, and then effectively spin our opponent around. It is fun. Reframing also helps. Instead of thinking, "Why do I have to deal with all these impossible people?" (and it is clear that some people *are* more impossible than others), we think, "Here is an opportunity to practice my new skills and see how I do." To the upset husband we say, "I know you have Jane's interest at heart and that you love her very much, *but* at this time I must do what she wants. In the long run, that will be very beneficial for her, which I know is what you want."

DEALING WITH FAMILY CONFLICT

In dealing with family members who disagree over goals and strategies, it is of critical importance to acknowledge the legitimacy of each person's position and reaction. Remember they all have different maps. It has been said that no two siblings have ever had exactly the same parents. They have all had different experiences of their family and tell themselves different stories (have very different memories). In trying to achieve some sort of consensus, it is important to help them focus on a superordinate goal—the welfare of the patient. If they cannot agree, then perhaps the practitioner's best judgment of the patient's needs has to prevail. If the practitioner has been supportive of the family and the patient, it is likely that they will agree on this. The practitioner takes responsibility because he or she has control of the treatment. Trying to modify family dynamics is an important challenge and requires creative interventions by the practitioner that are beyond the scope of this book.[1]

CONFRONTING THE PATIENT

There are times when a person's behavior goes beyond acceptable limits or causes a problem, making confrontation necessary. Under these circumstances, it is important to point out to the individual in what way the behavior is a problem (i.e., how it affects the practitioner, the staff, or the practice) and to suggest a specific correction. Sometimes this is enough, and the person will apologize and make the correction. More often, however, the person will become defensive and abusive and will refuse to discuss the issue. The way in which people react to being confronted with negative information about themselves that they do not wish to acknowledge (it is on their map, but they pretend it is not) or do not wish to change is usually stereotypical.[2] People will react as though they had been *zapped*. We can expect one of three potential behaviors in response to a *zap*: counterattack, retreat, or diffusion. The three responses work as follows:

Counterattack: "Really, Doctor, I want you to know that I have not been pleased with the way that you treated my mother. I think I will ask someone else to take over her care."

Retreat: "I'm sorry, Doctor, I don't have time to discuss it now (or ever). I'm late for an appointment."

Diffusion: "You think that I'm hard to deal with. My son has been giving me so much trouble lately. He has no plans for the future. What do you think is wrong with the current generation?"

Any of these reactions is typical for persons being *zapped*: that is, being confronted and having to deal with something they have been trying to avoid. When counterattacked by the "zappee," it is important for the practitioner to guard against feeling counterzapped but to switch to active listening and verbal aikido and then to repeat the original message. This is not as difficult as it sounds. When a negative reaction is expected, the practitioner can be prepared to handle it smoothly:

Fielding the counterattack: "Yes, I agree that sometimes you have not been pleased with my treatment choices, *but* you must cease bringing alcohol into the hospital."

The retreat: "Mr. Jones, I know you are in a hurry, *but* I want you to get that blood test done today."

The diversion: "Yes, I can see how frustrated you are with your son, *but* I must have your signed consent for this procedure, now."

And the combination of all three: "Mrs. Smith, I understand that you are angry because I sometimes don't call you back within a reasonable time frame and that your boss makes unreasonable demands on you at work and that you have to leave right now because your babysitter is unreliable, *but* I cannot continue to treat your diabetes if you will not take your medicine as prescribed."

The Ubiquitous Zap

Any time we confront others with something they really do not want to hear from us, it can be considered a *zap*. Zaps by definition are subjective experiences of the receiver, who will react (or rather overreact) in typical fashion. Recognizing this as normal, being prepared for it, and not reacting to the counterattack as if it were a zap are useful tactics. Retreats or diversions can also be expected (and must be accepted) before reiteration of the initial problem can be productive. Sometimes it is necessary to go through several rounds before finally being heard. This insight is helpful in all interpersonal situations involving conflict that must be addressed, in confronting others about unacceptable behavior, and particularly in dealing with difficult patients or their families.

TRAINING THE OFFICE STAFF

The office staff represents an important element of the environment that the patient experiences when coming to the practitioner for treatment. In fact, when calling to make an appointment or wanting to speak to the practitioner on the phone, the staff acts as the ultimate gatekeeper.

It is important that receptionists and nursing personnel become aware of the effects of stress on patients, as outlined in Chapter 2, and learn a few simple and effective interventions for managing patient interactions. For example, our receptionist complained that some patients are very difficult and demanding on the phone and that *they* should learn to be more cooperative. However, we know that people who are upset are often unreasonable. It is not useful to focus on the fact that they should not be that way; the reality is that they are. The question becomes "What can be done to make the person feel supported enough so that healthier responses can be expected? How can we deal with unreasonable patients without contributing to our own stress?"

Fielding Phone Calls

Sometimes when a practitioner has not returned a patient's call, for whatever reason, patients will become frustrated and abusive of the staff. Although we certainly do not condone this type of behavior, it is not useful for the receptionist to get upset and respond angrily to the patient. What is helpful is for the receptionist to make a supportive statement: "It must be difficult to have to stay home and wait for the doctor to call back, when you have so much to do (or you are feeling so bad)." "It must be hard when you are so worried about Nancy's fever to not be able to reach the doctor right away. Time passes so slowly when you're anxious, doesn't it?" This type of understanding response makes the patient feel supported, connected to another human being who acknowledges the reaction to the stress as being reasonable—which it is!

Creating Realistic Expectations

The second major thing that the staff must be encouraged to do is to help the patient set realistic expectations. It is of little value to get the patient off the phone by saying, "Yes, I'll tell the doctor to call you right away" when the doctor is not back from lunch, is solidly booked with patients all afternoon, and has to make hospital rounds after 5 o'clock, before going to an out-of-town medical society dinner at 7:30. Instead, it is better to say that the doctor will probably not be available to speak to the patient and ask if there a specific question that needs to be answered or if it can wait until morning.

It is important to specify when to expect the call back. The implication is that the patient's time is also valuable and that he or she has other things to do besides sitting by the phone and waiting for the practitioner to call back. If it becomes impossible for the practitioner to contact the patient within the agreed time period, someone else should call and inform the patient *when* the practitioner can be expected to be free.

We like to compare the experience of the patient to our own when we are phoning someone whose line is busy and we are put on hold. It is very reassuring to have the operator periodically break in and report that the line is still busy. The wait is no less interminable, but we know that we have not been forgotten. We have a sense of being acknowledged and still being connected. We need to ensure that patients do not feel forgotten and disconnected. By adopting these procedures, angry repeat calls from frustrated patients will be minimized

Patients in the Office

There are also potential problems related to patients in the office. Because of their particular personalities, the staff finds it extremely difficult to deal with certain patients. Although it is clear that these patients' personalities are not going to change, often their behavior can be managed more effectively. Objectively, these patients' problems may not be serious, but subjectively, their problems are disturbing their precarious equilibrium or they would not be coming to the office for help. The staff needs to understand that under stress patients are not at their best behavior. Unhappy patients may become demanding, unreasonable, angry, impatient, and even rude to the staff, although they often behave in a passive or ingratiating manner with the practitioner on whom they feel dependent.

The staff needs to be able to set reasonable limits, always acknowledging patients' rights to feel as they do and acknowledging their suffering but asserting the need to control their behavior. The receptionist must inform individuals reciting a laundry list of troubles, insults, and concerns that "I understand that it must be very difficult for you." "I can see how upset you are." "I can hear how angry and frustrated you feel, but . . . ." Direct acknowledgment of their suffering relieves patients of continued efforts to convince someone of their plight. Once they have successfully communicated that they are miserable, they will be more apt to be able to hear what others want.

The staff also needs to help patients set realistic expectations for the visit. It is better to say that there will be at least a half-hour wait, when the doctor is running behind schedule, than to say nothing, or worse yet, "The doctor will be right with you," when the doctor will not be right with them. When patients feel as though their comfort is a concern for others, it is more likely that they will be able to respond to the concerns of others.

Care for the Caring

The practitioner has a responsibility to support the office staff while encouraging concern for patients' well-being. It is important to be mindful of the fact that the staff also needs to feel competent and connected. Frequently acknowledging the contribution the staff is making to the supportive environment of the office will reinforce that practice: "I really appreciate the way you've handled Mrs. Brown. She must be very difficult for you to deal with." "You must really get tired of having to field all these phone calls when I have trouble getting back to these people in a timely fashion. I am impressed with the grace and skill you use." Positive reinforcement by definition increases the probability of the preceding behavior recurring.

RULES FOR PRACTITIONER SURVIVAL

We have been doing a great deal of preaching in this book regarding the need to take care of patients' psychological as well as physical needs. We are aware that in order for practitioners to follow through on these practices, their own psychological needs must be met. Since we try hard to be consistent, we will now provide a set of rules that the practitioner can apply to ensure personal psychological well-being. These rules were developed out of our teaching experience with residents. Here are the dozen we have found to be most helpful in practice.

Rule I: Do Not Take Responsibility for Things You Cannot Control.

The implication of this rule is that if we did not have control of the circumstances that created a situation, we do not have to take responsibility for the effect the situation has on others. The practical application of this rule is that when people complain about a situation over which *we* have no control, hence for which we are not responsible, we are able to empathize with their frustration, pain, or other discomfort without becoming *defensive*. Since it is clearly not our fault, we can sympathize with patients about the inflexibility of rules made by hospitals, their managed care organizations, or the government without feeling as though we are required to do anything except comfort the patient. It is a situation over which we have no control. Although the patient's anger may be expressed toward us, we know that it does not belong to us. This awareness allows us to gracefully duck and then support the patient. It is also important to remember that we are not responsible for creating the patient's disease. However, we may (or may not) be able to treat it effectively.

The corollary of Rule l is that we must take responsibility for what we can control—our own behavior. It is a given that in order to control our behavior, we must first be aware of it. We must also recognize our limits.

Rule 2: If You Do Not Take Care of Yourself, You Cannot Take Care of Others.

It is critical that practitioners become aware of their limits and tolerance for certain situations. When we find that we are going on *tilt*, it is imperative to take time out to center ourselves. Practitioners need to learn stress management techniques, build a support group, set realistic expectations for themselves, and set limits on the demands of others (gently, of course). Becoming overstressed impairs functioning. Once functioning is impaired, the outcome becomes questionable. This leads to Rule 3.

Rule 3: Trouble Is Easier to Prevent Than to Fix.

This concept needs little elaboration. Often one or two minutes spent explaining something or considering the consequences of a potential action can avoid extensive problems. Exploring potential outcomes and worst-case scenarios before the fact can ultimately save time and aggravation. Doing nothing is often better than doing something, especially when not all the data are in. Applying tincture of time when hasty action might precipitate an unstoppable process is an important option to consider.

Rule 4: When You Get Upset, Tune Into What Is Going on With You, and Go Through the Three-Step Process.

1. What am I feeling?
2. What do I want?
3. What can I do about it?

This effective strategy for getting in touch with and managing feelings and behavior was presented in Chapter 7. It is an important skill for the practitioner to apply personally. Whenever there is a sense of starting to approach *tilt*—feeling a strong sense of being internally pressured and clearly off balance—we recommend tuning in and labeling the experienced feeling. Is it anger, frustration, impatience, sadness, fatigue, or what? That is Step 1.

Step 2 requires getting in touch with what is actually wanted; for example, "I want the patients to stop being so demanding." "I want my receptionist to be better organized." "I want someone to take care of me, for a change." "I want someone to acknowledge that I am trying to do a good job."

Step 3 requires determining what one can do personally to accomplish what is desired. If we are more responsive to patients, they may actually become less demanding. The receptionist may need some support if this is an unusual style for him or her. However, if the disorganization is chronic and unremediable, the receptionist may need to be replaced. As far as getting someone to take care of us or acknowledge our accomplishments is concerned, we may have to learn to ask for what we want—and then to learn to accept it. Sometimes, there is *nothing* that we can do to get what we want. We cannot get it to stop raining on our parade. We cannot change the past or how someone else is feeling or reacting. We cannot stop people from dying. That brings us to Rule 5.

Rule 5: If the Answer to Step 3, Rule 4 Is "Nothing," Apply Rule 1.

Rule 1, of course, states that we should not take responsibility for things we cannot control. In this case, since there is nothing we can do to get what we want, we need to accept that fact. We do not beat up on ourselves for not being able to affect something over which we have no power. Given this realization and then recycling Rule 4 usually will result in feeling sad and wishing it was a more perfect world. Since we know there is nothing that we can do to make that happen, this usually results in a feeling of acceptance, smug satisfaction with becoming wiser, and an appreciation of ourselves and our ability to sort out feelings. It has been our experience that when we go through this process, there is generally a strong sense of taking control. By definition, this results in a sense of competence that is mutually exclusive to feeling overwhelmed. We are fixed!

We feel much better. This works for us just as it does for patients.

Rule 6: Ask for Support When You Need It—and Give Others Permission to Feel What They Feel.

This simple strategy affirms the importance of accepting both ourselves and others where we are, given our individual maps and stories. We all need support sometimes, and this need does not imply weakness. Although giving people permission to feel what they feel costs nothing, it is highly supportive. There is recognition of the fact that if they could feel differently, they would.

Rule 7: In a Bad Situation You Have Four Options.

1. Leave it.
2. Change it.
3. Accept it.
4. Reframe it.

This strategy was discussed at length in Chapter 8. We cannot underscore too strongly the empowering effect of learning to reframe situations. If there is nothing that we can do to change an uncomfortable circumstance, we can learn to give ourselves points for flowing with it, not upsetting ourselves, using the time to think about options for next time, or any other constructive attitude or behavior. Thus we can turn the situation into a successful learning experience. In any case, a way to program small wins must be found. The small win may simply be deciding not to complain, since it is futile and may only make others uncomfortable. Finding a constructive way to look at the circumstances (changing the story) so that it results in a positive personal outcome is the essence of reframing.

Rule 8: If You Never Make Mistakes, You Are Not Learning Anything.

Beating up on oneself for an honest, unintentional mistake is not constructive. Being human means that we cannot be perfect. If we do not *own* (or acknowledge) our mistakes, we cannot learn from them. Mistakes resulting from ignorance or fatigue can be reframed by recognizing that they need to be prevented. See Rule 3.

Rule 9: When a Situation Turns Out Badly, Identify the Choice Points and Then Decide What You Would Do Differently Next Time.

This rule needs little explanation. Again, the aim is to get something constructive from something that cannot be changed. If there is nothing that you would change, given a chance to replay the situation, it is important to acknowledge that there is no blame, since circumstances obviously did not work out as would generally be expected. However, it is usually a good idea to reexamine the original expectations and evaluate their innate reasonableness.

Rule 10: At Any Given Time, You Can Only Make Decisions Based on the Information You Have.

This was also discussed in Chapter 7. It is often useful to postpone decisions when the data are not in, to apply tincture of time, and to talk things through with supportive others.

Rule 11: Life Is Not Fair—and Life Is Not a Contest.

It is true, life really is not fair. Once we accept this fact, living becomes easier. We do not even have to feel guilty about talents and possessions that we have that less fortunate people lack. Moreover, life is not a contest. (Many people live as though it were.) It helps to realize that the important things—such as love, wonder, healing, or reaching one's potential—are on a different dimension from a zero-sum game. This is because the more we allow ourselves and others to be open to these experiences, the more resources become available for everyone. People who feel secure do not need to put other people down.

Rule 12: You Have to Start Where the Patient Is.

At any given time, people can only be where they are, given their maps and stories. They are reacting to their perceptions and doing the best they can. If they could be any different, they would be—and so would you. This does not mean that people cannot and do not change. People can and do change but only when they are ready to do so and when it is safe! Safe means being accepted "as is."

SUMMARY

In dealing with family members, power struggles must be avoided and verbal aikido is used to defuse opposition. People hear better when someone starts by agreeing with them. Relieving guilt is a therapeutic intervention. When having to confront patients or families, practitioners are warned to expect counterattacks, retreats, or diversions.

Training the office staff in supportive psychological strategies is effective, as is adopting enlightened expectations for oneself. It is important to be mindful of the fact that the staff also needs to feel competent and connected. Rules for practitioner survival based on our philosophy are presented.

REFERENCES

1. Doherty, W.J., & Baird, M.A. *Family Therapy and Family Medicine*. New York: Guilford Press, 1983.
2. Palmer, J.D. *Workshop on Improving Conflict Skills*. Unpublished paper, 1977.

CHAPTER 12

Anticipated Outcomes: Transcending Limitations

Incorporating therapeutic interventions into day-to-day primary care practice can enhance the experience of practitioners, patients, patients' families, the medical profession, and perhaps even society as a whole.

LIVING IN THE AGE OF ANXIETY

According to a recently published study that examined changes in anxiety and neuroticism during the years 1952 to 1993, Americans have shifted toward substantially higher levels of these negative emotional states.[1] Two meta-analyses found that both adults and children experienced significantly higher levels of anxiety during the latter half of the century. A striking finding was that the average American child in the 1980s reported more anxiety than child psychiatric patients did in the 1950s. In trying to explain these results, the researcher cited correlations with social indices, such as divorce and crime rates, and suggested that decreases in social connectedness and increases in environmental dangers might be responsible for the rise in anxiety.[1]

Another recent study highlights the importance of control as a factor in health.[2] When employees perceived they had control over their job responsibilities but did not have confidence in their problem-solving abilities or blamed themselves for bad outcomes, they were most likely to experience high levels of stress. Trying to practice good medicine within the limits set by government regulations and managed care corporations certainly has the potential for making practitioners feel a lack of control of their circumstances, as well as reducing their confidence in their ability to responsively manage patients' needs. We would encourage practitioners to find ways to reframe these problems positively as a challenge and growth opportunity.

A growing body of evidence suggests that our attitudes, both positive and negative, may be associated with physical health, mental health, and longevity.[3,4] In fact, researchers from the University of Kentucky found a strong association between written positive interpretations of circumstances in autobiographies and longevity of the authors 60 years later.[5] Psychologists have been seriously focusing on the need to understand and develop positive aspects of human nature and to foster optimism.[6] Resilience is cited as a quality leading to positive adaptation.[7] Realistic optimism, the tendency to maintain a positive outlook within situational constraints, increases the likelihood of desirable and personally meaningful outcomes.[8] Let us look at how this can be applied.

EFFECT ON THE PRACTITIONER

Clinicians practicing at this historical moment when the medical care delivery system is considered to be in a state of crisis must make a choice. Either they must accept the transformed medical paradigm, finding ways to integrate new techniques and new insights into their practices, or they can try to continue functioning according to the old medical model. If they choose to accept the enriched model, after an initial period of adjustment they are likely to achieve great personal satisfaction and constructive patient outcomes. On the other hand, if they stay with the old paradigm, they can expect large measures of frustration when both personal and patient outcomes turn out to be less than optimal.

Responding to a Changed Paradigm

Buckminster Fuller's work has cast out all doubt that we can any longer say, "It is fortunate that the Good Lord created the universe exactly divided into the traditional academic disciplines."[9] Just as biochemistry has bridged the gap between biology and chemistry, biophysics has bridged the gap between biology and physics and has much to teach us about immunology. The power of imagery to affect body processes is demonstrated daily through biofeedback. We know that how we think determines how we feel and that positive thoughts contribute to positive outcomes. We also know that how we think affects our physical reactions and that feeling powerful or helpless affects our ability to mobilize an effective immune response.[10] The most dangerous state, for our bodies, as well as for our minds, exists when we feel overwhelmed and demoralized.[11] All this puts a traditionally trained physician into a situation of great stress. Many absolutes that have formed the core of the practitioner's understanding are changing or have changed drastically. Having to adapt to rapidly changing circumstances precipitates a high level of stress. And how do people respond to overwhelming stress? Under extreme circumstances the following happens:

1. They intensify their usual psychological and social coping devices.
2. When these devices fail, they experience anger that must be suppressed (or even repressed) or else the sources of existing support will dry up more.
3. Next, they turn on themselves, blame themselves for not managing better, internalize their aggressive impulses, and develop feelings of guilt and depression.
4. Finally, they stop trying to cope; instead, they feel helpless and develop a variety of symptoms.

When people give up and stop trying to cope, the prescription is to provide support, thus gratifying dependency needs without undermining self-respect.

The strategies described in *The Fifteen Minute Hour* are designed to provide support for practitioners and patients alike. Our "cookbook" approach provides step-by-step instructions for applying effective techniques that can lead not only to improved patient care but also to enhanced satisfaction, increased income, and personal growth for the practitioner.

Applying a Therapeutic Strategy

For starters, the practicing professional can consider the following questions: How do you feel about what is going on in the medical care delivery system today? Or, how do you feel about how you are practicing medicine today? What do you want? In other words, how do you want to practice? And finally, what can you do about it? Translation: what changes do you have to make in order to be able to do this?

We recommend that the practitioner be very clear about the answers to these questions. If there is a desire to put things back to the way they were, unfortunately there is nothing that can be done about that. The road goes on. But if the desire is to keep up, be productive, and be successful, many strategies in this book will contribute to that goal, but only if put into practice.

Achieving Professional Success

Although many reimbursement systems actually create a financial incentive for keeping people well and preventing or limiting serious illness, we feel that regardless of what form payment may take, the practitioner has a moral obligation to practice preventive medicine. By monitoring stressful events in their patients' lives on an ongoing basis, problems may be caught earlier and at less complicated stages. Practitioners can experience great satisfaction when building a practice based on continuity of care, attention paid to lifestyle and other health-enhancing practices, and provision of anticipatory guidance. The most important payoff for the practitioner, however, may ultimately be the joy of participating meaningfully and contributing positively to the quality of patients' lives.

Personal Growth

The final payoff for practitioners adopting and using our therapeutic interventions on a day-to-day basis will be their own personal growth. By applying the principles outlined in this book to their own life situation, practitioners will feel empowered. It will become somewhat easier to juggle professional commitments, family obligations, and personal needs. Practitioners will develop their own sense of coherence and incorporate a rational, flexible, and far-sighted coping style.[12] In order to develop a coherent sense of identity, practitioners need to reflect on their feelings about their careers, relationships with both patients and colleagues, personal relationships, financial and security issues, relationships to the wider community, and ultimately the meaning of life.[13] Becoming aware of the feelings related to these issues, acknowledging wants, and deciding what strategies are available to meet reasonable expectations will lead to positive personal growth. As human beings, we may be organisms affected by our biology and demands from the environment, but we are also agents (subjects who act with intentionality), as well as spiritual beings with our place in the universe.

Moving Toward Self-Actualization

When needs for physical survival, security, acceptance, and achievement have been met, practitioners invariably approach that part of A.H. Maslow's hierarchy of needs identified as self-actualization.[14] Maslow pointed out that self-actualized people make full use of their talents, capabilities, and potentialities and develop to the full stature that they are capable of attaining.

Becoming self-actualized results in a more efficient perception of reality and more comfortable relations with it. Self-actualized people do not need to cling to positive illusions, nor do they need to cling to the familiar. They accept themselves, other people, and nature. They are relatively comfortable with the vague and indefinite, and the quest for truth assumes priority over the need for safety.[14] Self-actualized people develop an increased ability to be spontaneous and a code of ethics that is autonomous. Self-actualized people, like good practitioners, are more problem-centered than ego-centered. They exhibit a certain quality of objective detachment and have a need for privacy. They rely on their own interpretation of situations. In other words, they have an internal locus of control.

Other desirable qualities that Maslow[14] cites as characteristic of achieving self-actualization include a continued fresh appreciation of the richness of experience, profound interpersonal relationships, development of a democratic character structure, a sense that means are ends, creativeness, and a friendly sense of humor.

People are not born self-actualized. It is a state that is fostered by transcending difficulties and applying the type of therapeutic modalities we are advocating in this book. By using these techniques and teaching them to their patients, practitioners will inevitably be positively affected.

PATIENT FACTORS

Having discussed from a broad viewpoint the potential benefits likely to accrue to the practitioner who incorporates therapeutic interventions into the usual patient visit, let us now look at the potential cumulative effects on patients.

Supporting Health Rather Than Curing Disease

When dealing with patients' problems as outlined in this book, we do not suggest that the practitioner is curing in the traditional sense. It may well be that there is no such thing as a specific disease in the traditional sense or a specific cure. We are proposing that the patient's sense of well-being will be enhanced through the therapeutic interaction with the practitioner. This in turn will support the patient's own healing powers and allow the patient's immune system to function at a normal level of effectiveness.[15] Moreover, from a social perspective, when the patient feels empowered, the patient will behave in ways that will result in more productive interactions with other people.

We are not claiming that we have solutions to chronic problems that have eluded other well-meaning health professionals. Our approach is simply designed to maximize positive outcomes using easily learned, proven behavioral techniques that can be incorporated into the structure of a typical primary care visit and will capitalize on people's strengths.

For the final example to be presented in this book, let us look at the case of Emily M., the type of patient who is characterized by a really thick chart:

Emily M. is a 43-year-old female, with limited education, who came into the office two years previously complaining of chest pain. She brought prescriptions for 13 different medications prescribed by six different doctors. She had been hospitalized numerous times for extensive workups of multiple aches and pains for which she had gone to the emergency room and been admitted. Cardiologists, pulmonologists, gastroenterologists, orthopedists, otolaryngologists, and gynecologists had each run their battery of tests from computed tomography (CT) scans and colonoscopy to coronary catheterization, but no one was able to identify the origin of her symptoms. Each consultant added another drug to her regimen and referred her to the next specialist, until she had seen them all. Having run out of subspecialists, she came to the Family Practice Center.

History revealed that the onset of her various acute pains would correspond with arguments with her abusive, alcoholic, unemployed (disabled) husband. Overall, she presented with the affect and vegetative signs of depression. Dr. S.'s clinical impression was that Emily was suffering primarily from depressive and somatization disorders. He weaned her off all her medications except sublingual nitroglycerin, taught her relaxation techniques, and started her on an activating selective serotonin reuptake inhibitor (SSRI).

Emily was seen once per week for several months, during which time the emphasis was shifted away from her physical pains, to focus on her shattered living situation and family problems. A social worker and a women's self-help group were also involved in her case. Emily was given strict instructions to call the center when she experienced acute pain rather than going to the emergency room. During her regular office visits, Dr. S. attended to her physical complaints without lingering on them and then spent most of the 15-minute session listening to the precipitating factors and new stresses in her life. He offered support and acknowledged her suffering. Using the *BATHE* technique, he focused her on one problem during each session and wondered what Emily could do to improve matters. Intervals between visits were gradually increased until they were every four weeks. At this time, Emily showed up in the emergency room complaining of chest pain! No acute problem was found.

After that incident, regular visits were scheduled at intervals ranging from every two to every four weeks and Emily improved slowly but steadily. In contrast to the multiple admissions in each of the previous five years, she has remained out of the hospital for two years, except for one hospitalization for hypotonic bowel with partial obstruction at the time of her sister's death. Emily continues to be seen at regular intervals, and although her living situation is no better, she is functioning at a somewhat higher level than before.

In every case, our goals involve helping patients to achieve whatever potential is reasonable for them, *at this time*. For Emily to stay out of the hospital for two years is an enormous accomplishment. Although functioning marginally by society's standards, her current level of adaptation is nonetheless remarkable.

Patients' Realization of Their Own Potential

Rather than engaging patients in a relationship that fosters dependency, our support encourages them to maximize their own potential. We focus on their strengths and promote patients' awareness that they are exercising choices at all times, by pointing out that there are always options. It is the patients' responsibility to determine what these options are. Based on the information they have, we encourage them to make the best possible choice at any given time. The implication is that the practitioner and the patient are on the same side, that of the patient. It is through this partnership with the practitioner that patients achieve the confidence to act positively in their own interest.

Enhancing Health

It is generally accepted today that the patient's health is largely determined by what the patient does, that is, the type of lifestyle that the patient adopts, rather than what happens during a visit to a practitioner's office. It is not our intention to quarrel with this statement but rather to encourage the use of strategies and techniques to affect the patient's behavior or lifestyle in positive ways. When the practitioner provides the type of care that we are advocating, patients' satisfaction and subsequent compliance with practitioners' instructions will be greatly enhanced.[16]

When a patient is "somatizing" and the practitioner inquires about what is going on in the patient's life, some skeptics may still contend that an uninitiated patient may object to this change of focus. The following example presents one possible response:

Patient: "You're saying it's all in my mind?"
Practitioner: "No, not at all. What I think is that your body is telling you that you are under stress and really hurting."

We want patients to start listening to their bodies, to monitor themselves and become aware of the precursors to *tilt*. In this way they can ease the pressure on themselves without having to become sick.

In recent years, increasing numbers of patients are requesting that their physicians take a more active interest in their health and disease processes.[17] When patients are able to accept and utilize the support provided by the practitioner, we can expect positive health consequences. Patients' sense of well-being will be enhanced, resulting in increased resistance to stressors of all kinds. They may be less susceptible to infections of various sorts, less accident-prone, and able to handle life's problems in more constructive ways. They will become more aware of the impact of their own reactions on others and on the things that happen to them. This type of constructive adaptation can be expected to lead to better physical and mental health.[12]

Reducing the Incidence of Complications

The secondary prevention implicit in our model of practice is quite obvious. Since illness itself generally upsets the balance of psychosocial well-being for patients and their families, the benefits of preventing illness complications are clear. Patients are encouraged to engage their most constructive coping mechanisms, to recognize that they must lower their expectations, to feel supported, and to get their needs met on an ongoing basis rather than forcing the practitioner to manage a series of catastrophes. The trust generated by being cared for and cared about will enhance patients' sense of basic trust in the world (the sense of coherence), which can then be expected to result in improved health consequences.[12]

EFFECTS ON THE FAMILY

It is obvious from the above that improved patient functioning will trickle down to other family members.

Improved Relationships

When patients apply the personal strategies that we have outlined, their relationships within their families, their work settings, and the community in general will improve. People who feel personally powerful resist being exploited and also have less need to exploit others. Communication patterns that are open and direct allow problems to be handled in more productive ways. This may sound utopian, but we have seen the powerful effects of small wins in mobilizing patients. It is also amazing to see how support enables people to function in their healthy rather than their neurotic modes. When people engage their healthy maps of the world, their altered behavior and positive expectations for their relationships become self-fulfilling prophecies.

Countering Resistance

Of course, specific family dynamics, old conflicts, and competing and seemingly mutually exclusive opinions, agendas, and desires will complicate the effect of patients' newly acquired assertiveness. It is important to counsel patients that they may experience mixed reactions to changes they attempt to instigate. Although family interventions are beyond the scope of this book, we recognize that the patient is a member of a (family) system. Since every part of any system reciprocally affects every other part of the system, when the patient changes certain self-defeating behaviors, this will have significant effects on other family members. After some initial resistance, which may be quite painful, a new accommodation will be made, hopefully with healthier functioning for all.

Additional Consequences of Improved Patient Functioning

By encouraging patients to communicate more clearly and directly, they and other members of their family will have less need to manipulate each other by becoming sick or engaging in various other destructive behaviors. As patients apply the practical child management techniques that we have advocated, their children can be expected to grow up with a well-formed sense of security, self-respect, and self-esteem. These children will be comfortable solving problems and making choices. When faced with peer pressure to take on risks, they will automatically consider the worst case scenario and find ways to maintain friendships as well as their values. A benevolent circle, the essence of primary prevention, will be engaged. People who have an enhanced sense of health and well-being can be expected to treat other people with consideration and respect. Their stories about themselves, the world, and the other people in it will be positive. This can be expected to result in positive interactions with others. When a majority of people adopt this view, our society as a whole will benefit.

IMPLICATIONS FOR THE PROFESSION

The growing public dissatisfaction with the medical profession is no secret. Although the clamor for health care reform continues unabated, public dissatisfaction with the medical profession is not a new phenomenon.

Looking at the Historical Perspective

One of the major reasons for the establishment of the American Medical Association in the first place was general unhappiness with the then-existent state of medical care.[18] Over time, there has been some ebb and flow in the level of satisfaction with physicians. In the middle of this century, with all the advances being made by modern medicine, there was something akin to a flood tide, resulting in a national romance with the medical profession.[19] Those were the days when numerous medical television programs and motion pictures were popular. Everyone wanted someone like Dr. Marcus Welby (Robert Young) to be their own personal practitioner, with Dr. Ben Casey as his consultant. Unfortunately, the love affair has become history.

Currently, there seems to be more ebb than flow in the tide of satisfaction with the medical profession. We believe, as does Engel,[20] that much of this problem can be traced to the method of educating medical practitioners. As we stressed in Chapter l, the dualism that separates mind from body, and the reductionistic approach to medical problem solving, effectively isolates the disease from the patient, and the patient from the practitioner, when in reality they are inexorably linked.

Employing the New Paradigm

By adopting our therapeutic approach, the practitioner demonstrates the ability to integrate the psyche and the soma in a way that will convince the patient that this practitioner is interested not only in biological processes but also in the patient as a person. Physical health, mental health, and spiritual health are viewed as interrelated. There is no question that the practitioner must be eminently skilled in dealing with traditional biomedical problems, but to deal with only the organic is to deal incompletely with the patient or the problem. We know that by employing the techniques presented in this book, practitioners will be able to respond to more of the needs that are traditionally expressed by patients seeking treatment. This will improve the practitioner's effectiveness and image.

Among other benefits, the practitioner will be in a much better position in our increasingly litigious society. Patients do not sue practitioners with whom they have a relationship of mutual trust, respect, and caring.[21] Improved practitioner-patient communication is generally seen as the most effective method of preventing malpractice claims.[22] In fact, patients do not necessarily sue because there has been a bad outcome. Patients sue because they feel that the practitioner is not willing or able to explain to the patient or to the family how it happened. One of the authors (M.S.) designed an intensive course in *communication enhancement training* at the request of the Medical Inter-Insurance Exchange, the practitioner-owned malpractice carrier in New Jersey, teaching strategies to minimize or prevent these types of communication breakdowns.[23] *The Fifteen Minute Hour* was used as a text for this course. Norman Cousins has suggested that doctors who spend more time with their patients may have to spend less money on malpractice protection.[24] We agree, but we think that the *quality* of the time spent with the patient is more important than the quantity.

SOCIETAL IMPLICATIONS

Improving the health of the population has become a professed goal for our society. As stated in *Healthy People 2010: Understanding and Improving Health*,[25] good health means not only reducing unnecessary suffering, illness, and disability but also gaining an improved quality of life. The two major goals to be achieved are increasing the quality and years of healthy life and reducing health disparities among Americans. The primary care provider must play a critical role in the achievement of these goals.

Promoting Health

Healthy People 2010, which was developed through a collaborative process, presents a comprehensive set of national health objectives for the decade and is designed to measure progress over time.[25] There are 28 focus areas (or chapters), the first of which is "Access to Quality Health Services." The initial objective listed in that chapter is to increase the percentage of people with a usual primary care provider from a baseline of 77% to a 2010 target of 85%.[26] Clearly, this is expected to enhance the health of the population. Access to health care is also listed as one of the 10 leading health indicators. The other nine are physical activity, overweight and obesity, tobacco use, substance abuse, responsible sexual behavior, mental health, injury and violence, environmental quality, and immunizations.[27] Except for environmental quality perhaps, the type of practitioner-patient relationship we have been advocating can positively influence all these areas.

Helping People to Change Their Behavior

It is clear that health promotion strategies are largely related to lifestyle, meaning that the choices people make regarding their personal lifestyles have a powerful influence on their health status. The priorities for modification of lifestyles include the following: to increase physical activity and fitness; improve nutrition; diminish the use of tobacco, alcohol, and other drugs; engage in responsible sexual behavior; and decrease violent and abusive behavior. All these priorities can be achieved only through behavioral change. We have described many strategies in *The Fifteen Minute Hour* that practitioners can employ to empower patients to successfully change behaviors destructive to their health.

Focus on Mental Health

One of the major areas of focus of *Healthy People 2010* is the improvement of mental health in the population. Objectives include reducing the suicide rate for adults and adolescents, reducing the relapse rate for persons with eating disorders, and increasing the number of persons seen in primary health care who receive mental health screening and assessment.[28] Attention paid to patients' mental state in primary care settings is seen as promoting early detection and intervention for mental health problems.[29]

Specific objectives of *Healthy People 2010* include reducing the proportion of people aged 18 years and older with unrecognized depression from a baseline of 77% to 50%. Another objective is to increase the percent of people with recognized general anxiety disorders from 38% to 50%.[30] If all practitioners *BATHE*d their patients, these objectives would be easily achieved. Primary care providers are cited as the most likely choices of those who seek professional help for mental health problems. We want practitioners to feel comfortable providing it.

Health Communications

The section on health communications in *Healthy People 2010* acknowledges that patients have many opportunities to access health information.[31] Rapidly expanding sources of data and advice, such as the myriad web sites on the Internet, intersect with recent demands for more rigorous evaluation of all aspects of health care for evidence-based practices. Provider-patient communication is seen as a critical factor in the quality of the provider-patient interaction, patient behavior, and health outcomes. The development of practice guidelines to promote better provider-patient communication is suggested.[32] We heartily agree.

PUTTING HEALTH PROMOTION AND DISEASE PREVENTION INTO PRACTICE

As part of health maintenance functions, there is a clear directive for the primary care practitioner to screen for depression, anxiety, and stress-related problems and also to help patients manage their reactions to the events in their lives in the most constructive way possible. We have tried to outline how this can be done effectively and efficiently. At a minimum each patient can be *BATHE*d and given permission to feel whatever feelings are being experienced. Limited information can be provided regarding people's normal reactions to stress and loss. Specific suggestions are designed to help patients manage stress or other troubling situations effectively. Anticipatory guidance to minimize stress inherent in adjusting to expected transitions should become part of routine treatment, while the ongoing relationship with the primary care practitioner provides basic support. Practitioners must learn to ask questions that focus patients on their own strengths. Appendix A provides 12 effective questions and three excellent responses with which to start to accomplish these goals. The minimal investment in time used in employing these techniques will pay off with maximal therapeutic results. The process will also help practitioners transcend some of the frustrations inherent in the present health care delivery climate, connect meaningfully with their patients, and gain renewed personal and professional satisfaction.

SUMMING UP

A final question is whether the therapeutic interventions we have proposed really work. They always have. This type of therapy used to be called "moral treatment."

Moral treatment was practiced in the nineteenth century in America. This was before Sigmund Freud, Carl Jung, or Alfred Adler. It was also before the time of Wilhelm Wundt, Ivan Pavlov, B.F. Skinner, Neil Miller, Gregory Bateson, Fritz Perls, Martin Seligman, Alfred Bandura, Aaron Beck, and Albert Ellis. Long before any of us were even thought of, moral treatment was used to prevent, treat, and correct various causes of mental disorders. The therapeutic intervention consisted of creating a milieu in which the emphasis was on building up the self-esteem and self-control of patients through the judicious use of "rewards and punishments in the context of a strong emotional relationship with a doctor."[33]

We think it is a great idea for the twenty-first century and beyond, especially when we can incorporate the contributions of all the distinguished clinicians and theorists cited above. It will certainly enhance the physical, mental, and spiritual health of the patient as well as the health, happiness, and image of the practicing primary care practitioner.

REFERENCES

1. Twenge, J.M. The age of anxiety? Birth cohort change in anxiety and neuroticism, 1952–1993. *Journal of Personality and Social Psychology*, 2000, *79*(6), 1007–1021.
2. Schaubroeck, J., Jones, J.R., & Jia, L.X. Individual differences in utilizing control to cope with job demands: Effects on susceptibility to infectious disease. *Journal of Applied Psychology*, 2001, *86*(2), 265–278.
3. Fredrickson, B.L., & Levenson, R.W. Positive emotions speed recovery from the cardiovascular sequelae of negative emotions. *Cognition and Emotion*, 1998, *12*, 191–220.
4. Maruta, T., Colligan, R.C., Malinchoc, M., & Offord, K.P. Optimists vs pessimists: Survival rate among medical patients over a 30-year period. *Mayo Clinic Proceedings*, 2000, *75*, 140–143.
5. Danner, D.D., Snowdon, D.A., & Friesen, W.V. Positive emotions in early life and longevity: Findings from the Nun Study. *Journal of Personality & Social Psychology*, 2001, *80*(5), 804–813.
6. Seligman, M.E.P., & Csikszentmihalyi, M. Positive psychology: An introduction. *American Psychologist*, 2000, *55*, 5–14.
7. Masten, A.S. Ordinary magic: Resilience processes in development. *American Psychologist*, 2001, *56*(3), 227–238.
8. Schneider, S.L. In search of realistic optimism: Meaning, knowledge and warm fuzziness. *American Psychologist*, 2001, *56*(3), 250–263.
9. Fuller, R.B. *Synergistics.* New York: Macmillan Publishing Co., 1975.
10. Kiecolt-Glaser, J.K., Glaser, R., Gravenstein, S., Malarkey, W.B., & Sheridan, J. Chronic stress alters the immune response to influenza virus vaccine in older adults. *Proceedings of the National Academy of Sciences*, 1996, *93*, 3043–3047.
11. Ader, R., Felton, D.L., & Cohen, N. (eds.) *Psychoneuroimmunology*, 2nd ed. San Diego: Academic Press, 1991.
12. Antonovsky, A. *Health, Stress, and Coping.* San Francisco: Jossey-Bass, 1979.
13. Schmiedeck, R.A. The sense of identity and the role of continuity and confluence. *Psychiatry*, 1979, *43*, 157–164.

14. Maslow, A.H. Self-actualizing people: A study of psychological health. *Personality*, 1950, *symposium 1*, 11–34.

15. Glaser, R., Rabin, B., Chesney, M., Cohen, S., & Natelson, B. Stress-induced immunomodulation: Implications for infectious diseases? *Journal of the American Medical Association*, 1999, *281*, 2268–2270.

16. Ley, P. Satisfaction, compliance and communication. *British Journal of Clinical Psychology*, 1982, *21*, 241–254.

17. Quill, T.E., & Brody, H. Physician recommendations and patient autonomy: Finding a balance between physician power and patient choice. *Annals of Internal Medicine*, 1996, *125*, 763–769.

18. Starr, P. *The Social Transformation of American Medicine*. New York: Basic Books, 1984, p. 424.

19. Lieberman, J.A., III. Family medicine and the aging patient: Clinical and educational issues. *New Jersey Family Practitioner*, 1984, *8*, 28–33.

20. Engel, G.L. The clinical application of the biopsychosocial model. *American Journal of Psychiatry*, 1980, *137*, 535–544.

21. Krause, H.R., Bremerich, A., & Rustemeyer, J. Reasons for patients' discontent and litigation. *Journal of Cranio-Maxillo-Facial Surgery*, 2001, *29*(3), 181–183.

22. Shapiro, R.S., Simpson, D.E., Lawrence, S.L., Talsky, A.M., Sobocinski, K.A., & Schiedermayer, D.L. A survey of sued and nonsued practitioners and suing patients. *Archives of Internal Medicine*, 1989, *149*, 2190–2196.

23. Stuart, M.R. *Communications Enhancement Training: Essential Skills to Lower the Risk of Malpractice Suits*. Seminar. Twenty-third Annual STFM Spring Conference, Seattle, May 1990.

24. Cousins, N. *The Healing Heart*. New York: W.W. Norton & Co., 1983, p. 162.

25. U.S. Department of Health and Human Services. *Healthy People 2010*, 2nd ed. With *Understanding and Improving Health* and *Objectives for Improving Health*. 2 vols. Washington, D.C.: U.S. Government Printing Office, November 2000.

26. U.S. Department of Health and Human Services. *Objectives for Improving Health*, p. 1–20.

27. U.S. Department of Health and Human Services. *Healthy People 2010*, 2nd ed. With *Understanding and Improving Health* and *Objectives for Improving Health*. 2 vols. Washington, D.C.: U.S. Government Printing Office, November 2000, p. 24.

28. U.S. Department of Health and Human Services. *Healthy People 2010*, 2nd ed. *Objectives for Improving Health*, p. 18–11.

29. U.S. Department of Health and Human Services. *Objectives for Improving Health*, p. 18–16.

30. U.S. Department of Health and Human Services. *Objectives for Improving Health*, p. 18–17.

31. U.S. Department of Health and Human Services. *Objectives for Improving Health*, p. 11–7.

32. U.S. Department of Health and Human Services. *Objectives for Improving Health*, p. 11–18.

33. Freedman, A.M., Kaplan, H.I., & Sadock, B.J. *Modern Synopsis of Comprehensive Textbook of Psychiatry II*, 2nd ed. Baltimore: The Williams & Wilkins Co, 1976, p. 22.

Twelve Good Questions and Three Good Answers for All Seasons

Questions That Have Therapeutic Value

1. How do you feel about that?
2. What troubles you the most?
3. How are you handling that?
4. What are you feeling right now?
5. What do you want?
6. What can *you* do about that?
7. What are your options?
8. What is the best thing that can happen?
9. What is the worst thing that can happen?
10. What is in it for you?
11. What does it mean to you?
12. What, specifically, were you hoping I would do?

Responses That Have Therapeutic Value

1. That must be very difficult for you.
2. I can understand *that* you would feel that way.*
3. Under the circumstances, I am sure that you (he, she, they) did the best you (he, she, they) could!

---

*Not to be confused with "I understand how you feel" or "I know how you feel," which are not recommended since they may lead to arguments. No one can actually know how another is feeling.

Recommended Books for Patients

Anxiety and Depression

Burns, D. *Feeling Good.* New York: Morrow, 1980.

Assign this book, a few chapters at a time, to all your depressed patients. It takes a sensible and effective approach to managing the symptoms of depression. There are inventories, exercises, and clear explanations. With your encouragement patients will benefit enormously.

Jeffers, S. *Feel the Fear and Do It Anyway.* New York: Fawcett Columbine, 1987.

This is an absolutely delightful, practical manual to help patients overcome the fears that limit their lives. An easy-to-read and easy-to-apply volume, it contains many exercises that can lead to insights. Patients can choose to work on certain sections and report their progress to the practitioner.

McKay, M., Davis, M., & Fanning, P. *Thoughts and Feelings: Taking Control of Your Moods and Your Life.* Oakland, Calif.: New Harbinger Publications, 1997.

This is a workbook of cognitive-behavioral techniques effective for worry control, coping with panic, and overcoming phobias. Patients can also learn to relax, stop unwanted thoughts, change habits, and adjust limited thinking patterns.

Young, J.E., & Klosko, J. *Reinventing Your Life.* New York: Plume, 1994.

This book presents evidenced-based cognitive techniques for helping patients make major changes in their approach to handling problems. It can facilitate long-lasting improvements from self-defeating patterns of behavior.

Stress Management

Davis, M., Eshelman, E.R., & McKay, M. *The Relaxation & Stress Reduction Workbook,* 5th ed. Oakland, Calif.: New Harbinger Publications, 2000.

This is a complete guide to relaxation techniques that includes chapters on breathing, meditation, visualization, stopping stressful thoughts, time management, nutrition, and physical exercise. It is a particularly effective self-help manual, especially if used with a clinician's supervision. New Harbinger Publications has a whole catalog of self-help materials focusing on every imaginable topic from communication skills (*Messages*) and eating disorders (*The Deadly Diet*) to lifetime weight control (*The Body Image Workbook*).

Assertiveness Training

Alberti, R.E., & Emmons, M. *Your Perfect Right*, rev. ed. San Luis Obispo, Calif.: Impact Press, 1974.

This is considered the classic on assertiveness training. It is sensibly written and easy to follow.

Smith, M.J. *When I Say No, I Feel Guilty*. New York: The Dial Press, 1975.

This book presents assertiveness training with humor and great examples. Let patients read and enjoy, and then assign them exercises to put into practice.

Parenting Guidance

Faber, A., & Mazlish, E. *How to Talk So Kids Will Listen, How to Listen So Kids Will Talk*, 20th ed. New York: Avon Books, 1999.

This little paperback is based on the work of Chaim Ginott, M.D., and is filled with cartoons and practical suggestions. It will make parents feel as though they have a wise and loving advisor always at hand to help them to deal with normal developmental issues in good-humored ways.

Gordon, T. *P. E. T.: Parent Effectiveness Training*. New York: Crown Publishers Group, 2000.

This classic still dispenses very good advice. It helps parents to set limits and makes them feel competent in their role.

Satir, V. *The New Peoplemaking*. Palo Alto, Calif.: Science and Behavior Books, 1988.

Virginia Satir's philosophical approach is designed to maximize self-esteem in all members of the family. A lovely book to read and enjoy, it nonetheless casts light on the dynamics of healthy and dysfunctional families. It should be available in all public libraries.

Dealing With Loss

Jewett, C.L. *Helping Children Cope With Separation and Loss*. Boston: The Harvard Common Press, 1982.

This book gives simple techniques for adults to use to help children who experience losses. It includes good background material on stages of grief and effects on children, as well as practical advice from how to tell children that something dreadful has happened, through the shock and denial, to the anger and depression that can be expected to follow. It also gives excellent suggestions for dealing with difficult situations brought on by death, separation, divorce, hospitalizations, major moves, or other traumatic events for children.

Kusher, H.S. *When Bad Things Happen to Good People*. New York: Avon Books, 1981.

This is a wonderful book to recommend for people who are dealing with tragedy. It is a comforting book that can help patients make sense out of their suffering.

For Everyone

Blanchard, K., & Johnson, S. *The One Minute Manager*. New York: Berkley, 1983.

This book is not just for managers. It helps focus people on what is essential: goals, praise, and complaints. These need to be concisely formulated and communicated clearly. This little book can help patients feel competent and connect with others in positive ways.

Index